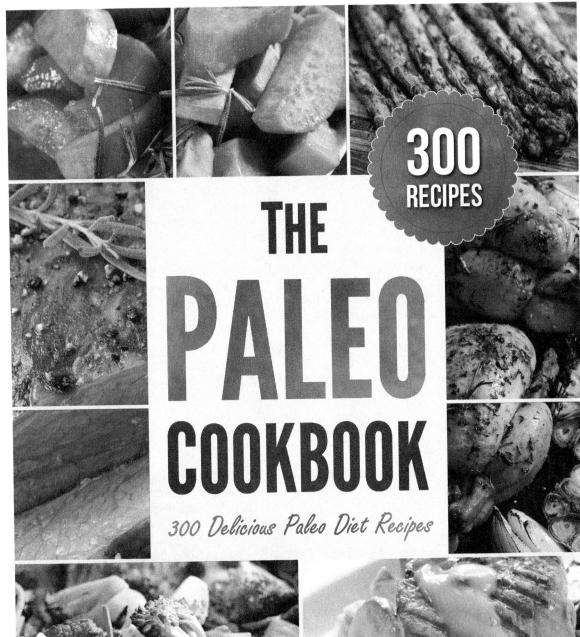

THE
PALEO
COOKBOOK

300 Delicious Paleo Diet Recipes

300 RECIPES

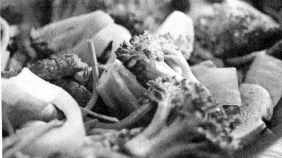
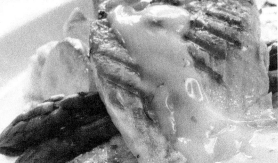

CONTENTS

Contents

WHAT IS THE PALEO DIET?

The Paleo diet has become incredibly popular in the past few years, leading many people to assume that it's a new way of eating. In reality, the Paleo diet has been around for almost forty years.

How the Paleo Diet Came About

In 1975, a gastroenterologist named Dr. Walter Voegtlin published a book called *The Stone Age Diet*. In the book, he documented how he treated patients with a diet that replicated the eating patterns of people during the Paleolithic era. The diet prescribed consuming large quantities of animal fats and proteins and very small quantities of carbohydrates. Dr. Voegtlin reported that his patients, who suffered from disorders such as Crohn's disease and irritable bowel syndrome, showed significant health improvements when following the diet.

Unfortunately, *The Stone Age Diet* didn't make much headway with the public. At that time, almost everyone believed that a low-fat, low-calorie diet was the only healthy way to eat.

An Ancient Diet for Modern Times

Ten years later, however, Dr. S. Boyd Eaton and Dr. Melvin Konner published a paper in *The New England Journal of Medicine* that supported Dr. Voegtlin's research and that received a lot of attention from the medical community and the media. The popularity of their paper on the Paleolithic era diet led to the publication of their book, *The Paleolithic Prescription: A*

Program of Diet & Exercise and a Design for Living. This book established the principles most variations of the Paleo diet people follow today.

The book explained the way our Paleolithic ancestors ate and why that nutritional lifestyle was such a healthy one. The most important thing the authors accomplished was to make the ancient diet suitable for modern times. The book laid out the nutritional content of the original Paleolithic diet and then showed readers how to get that nutritional profile from modern and widely available foods. It was an adaptable way to eat like our ancestors, and it paved the way for today's Paleo diet phenomenon.

The Paleo Diet for You, the Modern Cave-Dweller

There are several versions of the Paleo diet around today; these versions generally differ in terms of how strictly they follow the eating patterns of our Paleolithic ancestors. The Paleo diet described in this book is a version that intends to closely duplicate the nutritional makeup of a Paleolithic diet without being unrealistic, difficult or complicated. You'll reap the health and weight loss benefits of the Paleo diet without having to turn your entire lifestyle inside out or spend time searching for exotic ingredients. You'll be practicing a diet that is moderate in its approach, but you will likely see incredible results.

What the Paleo Diet Looks Like

The Paleo diet is designed to duplicate the results and benefits of our pre-agricultural diet without duplicating the diet's prehistoric methods. While there are a few Paleo followers who do literally hunt, gather or forage all of their food, most people don't have the motivation or time for that level of authenticity. Fortunately, we can achieve the same Paleolithic results with foods readily available to us in grocery stores, health foods stores and farmers markets.

The Paleo diet food pyramid is an inverted version of the one that used to be recommended by the USDA. Meats, eggs and seafood make up the majority of the day's calories, followed by fats from plant foods, fruits and vegetables, and then nuts and seeds. The Paleo diet is a high-protein/low-carbohydrate diet.

In Chapter 2, we go into more detail on what you'll be eating from each food group and also give you a specific list of allowed (and disallowed) foods. For now, we'll cover the basics.

What Is Not on Your Paleo Plate?

The Paleo diet is effective not only because of what you eat, but also because of what you don't eat. Changing the components and proportions of your diet is only half of the Paleo plan. The other half involves eliminating foods that can slow your metabolism, encourage blood sugar problems and fat storage, and slow digestion. These eliminated foods include processed foods, alcohol, grains, legumes and sugar.

Processed Foods

Fast food, frozen meals and store-bought sweets and snacks are not a part of the Paleo diet and should be avoided.

Grains

Grains, including all breads, pasta, rice, oats and barley, are agricultural products; you are embarking on a pre-agricultural diet. Later in this chapter, we'll explain in greater detail why grains are specifically off-limits.

Legumes

As with grains, legumes such as beans, peas, soy and soy derivatives are agricultural products and are therefore off-limits. we'll explain the specific risks to your health that these foods pose later in this chapter.

Sugar

One of the remarkable things about the Paleo diet is the impact it can have not only on lowering blood sugar levels, but also on decreasing your risk of developing diabetes and metabolic syndrome. In part, this is because sugars are eliminated on the Paleo diet. It is also very important to avoid substituting artificial sweeteners for sugar. You can, however, use honey in moderation, as it was likely a part of the ancestral diet. Chocolate may be consumed, but choose unsweetened and dark varieties.

What Is on Your Paleo Plate?

Meats, Eggs and Seafood

This food group is where you will get most of your calories. All meat, fish, shellfish, mollusks, and eggs are allowed, but there are some guidelines for choosing the right foods for the best results. The most important thing is that these foods are of high quality and are prepared with Paleo-approved ingredients.

Fats from Plant Sources

These sources include olives and olive oil, avocadoes (which are a fruit but serve as a fat), and nuts and seeds (which are described in detail in the next section). Since butter is a dairy product and does not improve your heart health, it should be avoided when cooking or preparing foods; use pure olive oil for cooking and grapeseed oil or extra virgin olive oil for uncooked dressings.

Nuts and Seeds

Nuts and seeds were a big part of the Paleolithic-era diet. All nuts are allowed, with the exception of peanuts, which are a legume. Seeds are allowed, including flax seeds, sunflower seeds, pumpkin seeds, sesame seeds and others. If you are frightened by the idea of giving up pasta and rice, the good news is that quinoa is allowed. Not only is quinoa a seed, but it also makes a great substitute for rice, pasta, oats, barley and other grain foods.

Fruits and Vegetables

The fruits allowed on the Paleo diet are those that would have been readily available (foraged) in the pre-agricultural era. These foraged fruits include berries, such as cranberries, raspberries, strawberries and blueberries. Tree fruits are also a mainstay of the Paleo diet; they include citrus fruits, apples, peaches, plums, cherries, nectarines and pears.

Choose vegetables that can be foraged in the wild. This eliminates most root vegetables, such as potatoes, sweet potatoes, carrots and parsnips, but includes wild root vegetables. Foraged vegetables include lettuces and leafy greens, tomatoes, peppers, squash and zucchini.

Condiments

Some condiments are allowed, but they should be limited to those that do not contain sugar or any of the forbidden ingredients. Ketchup, for example, is not allowed; mustard, on the other hand, is made from seeds and usually does not contain added sugar. In general, try to rely on herbs and spices rather than condiments.

Beverages

Allowed beverages include pure fruit and vegetable juices, but they should be unsweetened versions and consumed in moderation. Water should be your primary beverage. Tea and coffee are acceptable on the Paleo diet, as long as you use almond milk to lighten them, rather than dairy milk. Alcohol should be consumed only occasionally, and always choose gluten-free beer or hard ciders if you want to imbibe. Some recipes in this book call for organic wines, as they don't contain sulfites or other additives.

2

EGGS AND BREAKFASTS

Grain-Free Pancakes

Nut butter and eggs make fine substitutes for flour in these pancakes. The pancakes cook up light, flavorful and slightly creamy, and with 9.5 grams of protein per serving, they'll keep you full for hours. Drizzle them with a bit of honey for a sweet taste if necessary, but remember to watch your sugar intake—especially for breakfast.

- 4 ripe bananas
- 4 large eggs
- ½ cup nut butter

- Freshly ground black pepper, to taste
- 2 teaspoons olive or coconut oil

Place the bananas in a large bowl and mash them with a fork until smooth. Beat the eggs in a separate bowl until frothy. Add them to the bananas.

Add the nut butter and mix well until creamy and smooth. Season with freshly ground black pepper.

Heat the olive oil in a skillet or on a griddle. Pour ¼ cup pancake batter for each pancake onto the griddle or skillet. Cook pancakes for 2 minutes and then flip with a spatula. Cook an additional 2 minutes, or until the pancakes are golden brown.

Serves 4

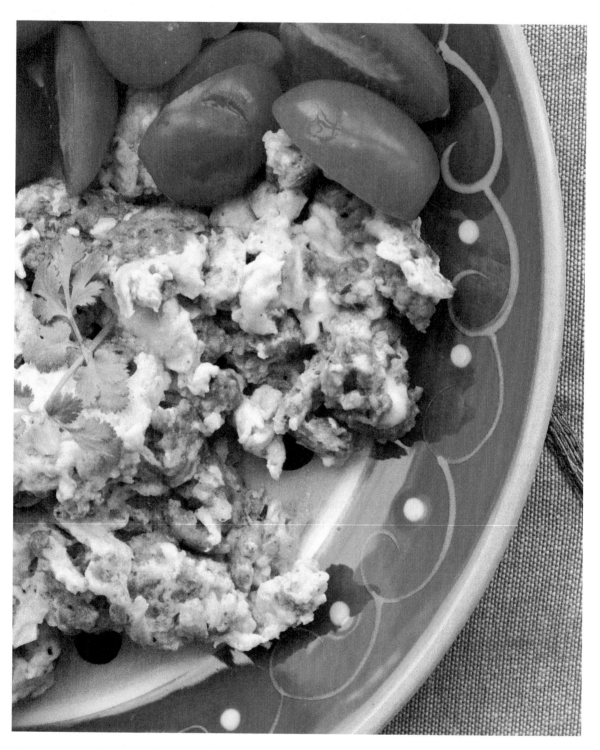

Mexican Veggie Scramble

Mexican Veggie Scramble

Loaded with veggies and high-protein eggs, this dish is filling and easy to make, but also delicious. Garnish with avocado and your favorite salsa for a south-of-the-border meal you won't forget. Think you'll miss the cheese? You may be surprised.

- 1 tablespoon olive or coconut oil
- ½ small onion, chopped
- ½ green bell pepper, diced
- ½ pound minimally processed chorizo sausage, cooked and crumbled
- 4 large eggs, beaten
- Freshly ground black pepper, to taste
- Sliced avocado, for garnish
- Prepared salsa, for garnish

In a medium non-stick skillet, heat the oil over medium heat. Add the onion and bell pepper and cook until soft. Add the sausage and eggs and stir continuously until eggs are cooked through. Season with freshly ground black pepper.

To serve, divide between plates and top with avocado and salsa.

Serves 2

Zesty Breakfast Salad

Salad for breakfast? Sure! This fruit and nut salad has a citrus dressing that will wake up your taste buds and get you ready for the day. Hard-boiled eggs and bacon add protein to keep you full for hours.

Salad:
- 2 cups baby spinach
- 1 large egg, hard-boiled and sliced into ½-inch chunks
- 1 strip uncured, nitrate-free bacon, cooked and crumbled
- 1 Clementine orange, peeled and quartered
- ½ cup dried cranberries or cherries
- ½ cup macadamia nuts, black walnuts, or pecans
- Freshly ground black pepper, to taste

Dressing:
- 1 tablespoon honey
- 1 teaspoon dry mustard
- ¼ cup red wine vinegar
- Juice of one orange
- 1 teaspoon onion, finely minced
- 1 cup olive oil
- Zest of 1 orange

Toss the spinach, eggs, bacon, orange quarters, dried cranberries, and nuts together in a bowl. Season with freshly ground black pepper.

Whisk the dressing ingredients together in a bowl for 30 seconds, or until the dressing becomes thick and creamy.

Divide on to 2 plates, and drizzle dressing over salad.

Serves 2

Paleo Breakfast Burrito

If you're craving a breakfast burrito, you'll love this Paleo-adapted recipe. Instead of a tortilla filled with eggs and meat, the eggs become the tortilla, leaving you with the same flavors rolled up into a tasty, easy to eat breakfast that will leave you full for hours. For best results, use a medium-sized skillet so that your eggs are super thin and easy to wrap. You'll never miss out on the high-carb tortilla!

- ¼ pound grass-fed ground beef
- 1 teaspoon cumin
- 1 teaspoon garlic powder
- 1 teaspoon onion powder
- 3 large eggs, beaten
- 1 tablespoon olive or coconut oil
- ½ small red onion, finely chopped
- Freshly ground black pepper, to taste
- Fresh cilantro, chopped, for garnish
- Prepared salsa for serving

Brown the beef in a skillet over medium heat. Once the meat is no longer pink, add the onion and season with the cumin, garlic powder, and onion powder. Set aside.

Whisk eggs in a small mixing bowl. Heat oil in a medium skillet over medium-low heat. Add the eggs in a thin, even layer and cook for about 6 minutes. Carefully flip the eggs over and continue cooking until done. Season with freshly ground black pepper. Carefully slide the eggs onto a plate. Top with the seasoned meat, cilantro, and salsa.

Serves 1

High-Protein Frittata

This is an easy breakfast dish that is loaded with protein. You can customize it to your liking, so use whatever veggies you like or have in your fridge. This is a great way to use up leftovers.

- 1 tablespoon olive or coconut oil
- ½ small onion, chopped
- ½ cup mushrooms, sliced
- 2 cups baby spinach leaves
- 8 large eggs
- Freshly ground black pepper, to taste
- 4 strips of uncured, nitrate-free bacon, cooked and crumbled

Preheat oven to 350 degrees F. Heat a large ovenproof skillet over medium heat and add the oil and vegetables. Sauté until tender. Remove from skillet and set aside.

Beat eggs in a large bowl and add the cooked vegetables. Season with freshly ground black pepper. Pour mixture into the skillet and put in the oven. Bake for 12 to 15 minutes or until eggs are firm to the touch.

Top with crumbled bacon and serve immediately.

Serves 4

Eggs Benedict Paleo Style

While this might not be the traditional version of eggs Benedict, you'll love this grain-free version that is as good for you as it tastes. Once you try it, you'll never want to go back to the old version again!

- ½ medium avocado
- 2 tablespoons lemon juice
- 1 clove garlic
- 1 large egg
- 1 tomato slice
- 2 slices uncured, nitrate-free bacon, cooked and crumbled
- Freshly ground black pepper, to taste

Put the avocado, lemon juice, and garlic in a food processor and process until smooth and creamy.

Poach the egg in a pot of simmering water until done, about 4 minutes.

To serve, place the egg on top of the tomato slice and top with the avocado sauce and bacon. Season with freshly ground black pepper.

Serves 1

Everything Omelet

An omelet is a fast and easy way to have a quick and filling breakfast that seems like a meal at your favorite breakfast spot. This version uses a variety of meats and veggies, but the beauty of this dish is that you can use whatever you have on hand for excellent results. If you have the time, you can leave it open for a frittata-like dish.

- 3 large eggs
- 1 tablespoon olive or coconut oil
- ½ small onion, chopped
- ½ cup broccoli, steamed
- 2 slices uncured, nitrate-free bacon, cooked and crumbled
- 2 minimally processed sausage links, cooked and chopped
- Freshly ground black pepper, to taste

Beat the eggs in a small bowl. Heat a small non-stick skillet over medium heat and add the oil.

Pour the eggs into the pan and allow to cook for 1 minute. Add the veggies and meat to one side and carefully fold the other side over the top of it. Cook until eggs are cooked through. Season with freshly ground black pepper.

Slide onto a plate and serve garnished with more bacon, if desired.

Serves 1

Egg Casserole for One

Sometimes you are in the mood for a delicious breakfast casserole filled with eggs, veggies, and breakfast meats, but you don't have the time or need for a full-fledged kitchen marathon. If this is the case, this recipe fits the bill. It's fast, easy, and doesn't leave you with leftovers you can't eat. For two, simply double the recipe and divide between two ramekins, or use a casserole dish if you're serving more than one. Either way, you'll love it!

- 2 large eggs
- 2 broccoli florets, finely chopped
- ¼ small zucchini, chopped
- ¼ small onion, chopped
- 5 spinach leaves, chopped

- 2 slices uncured, nitrate-free bacon, cooked and crumbled
- 1 tablespoon olive or coconut oil
- Freshly ground black pepper, to taste

Preheat oven to 350 degrees F. Beat eggs in a small bowl and mix in the veggies and bacon. Season with freshly ground black pepper.

Grease a single-serve ramekin with oil and pour the egg mixture in. Bake for 15 to 20 minutes until the top is lightly browned. Serve immediately.

Serves 1

Poached Eggs and Root Vegetable Hash

Root vegetables are high in fiber and flavor, and are a unique twist on the veggies you usually see with your morning eggs. Warm and crispy, they make a great substitute for potatoes, with fewer carbs and a lot more nutrients.

- 1 large beet, peeled and chopped
- 1 medium turnip, peeled and chopped
- 1 small onion, chopped
- 2 tablespoons olive or coconut oil
- 1 sprig fresh rosemary, finely chopped
- Freshly ground black pepper, to taste
- 1 clove garlic, minced
- 4 large eggs

Preheat oven to 400 degrees F. Toss veggies in the oil and lay on a single-layer sheet pan. Sprinkle on chopped rosemary. Season with freshly ground black pepper. Roast for about 15 minutes, remove from oven, and add the garlic. Roast for 10 more minutes, or until crispy around the edges.

While the veggies are cooking, poach eggs in a pot of simmering water, until just cooked.

To serve, divide the root vegetables between two plates and top with two eggs. Serve immediately.

Serves 2

Mini Egg Casseroles

These mini egg casseroles are quick to make and easy to take. They rely on sautéed veggies for their flavor, without the addition of cheese. Freeze them for later and microwave them on low for 30 seconds when you're ready to use them. That way, you can have a quick and filling breakfast (or snack) anytime you want!

- ½ cup onion, minced
- ½ cup red bell pepper, chopped
- 2 strips uncured, nitrate-free bacon, crumbled
- 8 large eggs, beaten
- 1 teaspoon dill
- Freshly ground black pepper, to taste

Preheat the oven to 350 degrees F. Spray one muffin pan with cooking spray. Spray a skillet with cooking spray as well.

Sauté the onions and bell pepper in the skillet over medium heat. This extra step really makes the difference in flavor in this recipe.

Combine the onions and bell pepper in a bowl with the remaining ingredients. Season with freshly ground black pepper.

Pour ½ cup egg mixture in each muffin tin. Bake for 10 to 12 minutes, or until set and slightly golden.

Serves 4

Scrambled Eggs with Lox

Traditionally, lox is served with high-carb bagels and cream cheese. While these may taste good, neither fits in a Paleo lifestyle. This version uses high-protein eggs and sliced tomatoes for a healthier version that you'll find just as tasty as the original. Smoked whitefish works well here too for a change of pace once in a while.

- 1 tablespoon olive or coconut oil
- ½ small red onion, diced
- 3 large eggs
- 2 ounces smoked salmon, chopped
- Freshly ground black pepper, to taste
- 1 large tomato, sliced
- 1 teaspoon capers
- 1 tablespoon fresh parsley, chopped

Heat oil in a medium skillet and add the onions. Cook until soft.

Beat the eggs in a small bowl and add the salmon. Season with freshly ground black pepper. Pour egg mixture over onions and scramble until cooked through.

To serve, top the tomato slices with the eggs and garnish with capers and parsley.

Serves 1

Chicken with Sweet Potato Hash Browns

It's hard to find a breakfast on the Paleo plan that doesn't include eggs, but this is one. You can serve it with eggs if you'd like, of course, but this dish stands on its own pretty well. Dark-meat chicken works nicely here, but use whatever you have on hand—it will still be delicious. The sweet potatoes make an excellent substitute for traditional greasy and high-carb hash brown potatoes.

- 2 sweet potatoes, peeled and diced into small pieces
- 2 tablespoons olive oil
- ½ small onion, diced
- 4 chicken thighs, cooked, meat pulled off bones and chopped or shredded
- 1 teaspoon each, dried thyme and oregano
- Freshly ground black pepper, to taste

Either in a microwave or steamer, steam sweet potatoes until tender and easily pierced with a fork. Divide in half and mash one half with a fork or potato masher.

In a large skillet, heat oil over medium-high heat. Add onion and cook until tender. Add chicken and spices, except pepper, and combine.

Add both sweet potato mixtures to the pan and combine the mixture thoroughly. Season with freshly ground black pepper.

Continue cooking until browned on the bottom, then flip to cook the other side until browned. Break up into small pieces and serve.

Serves 4

Paleo Muffins

There's a reason why muffins are popular breakfast items: They're easy to grab and go. Unfortunately, what you gain in convenience, you usually give up in health content. Not so with these muffins. Loaded with veggies, they are easy to whip up and you can keep them around for those mornings when you just need something you can grab as you're headed out the door. No more worrying about indulging in high-carb muffins when you've got this high-protein version on hand.

- 1 teaspoon olive or coconut oil
- ½ medium onion, chopped
- 1 cup broccoli, finely chopped
- ½ green bell pepper, diced
- ½ red bell pepper, diced
- 8 large eggs
- Freshly ground black pepper, to taste

Preheat oven to 400 degrees F. Grease a muffin tin with oil. Mix veggies in a large bowl and divide equally among muffin tins.

Beat eggs in a large bowl. Season with freshly ground black pepper. Pour mixture over veggies in the muffin pan.

Bake for 15 to 20 minutes, or until tops are browned. Loosen with a knife around the edges and cool before serving.

Makes 1 dozen

Paleo Huevos Rancheros

This popular egg dish is usually served with corn tortillas and beans, but once you try this version, you'll be surprised by how tasty it can be without those high-carb additions. You don't need those energy-sucking carbs for breakfast! This makes a fabulous brunch option as well.

- 1 tablespoon olive or coconut oil
- 2 cloves garlic, minced
- 1 red bell pepper, chopped
- ½ small onion, diced
- 1 jalapeño pepper, minced
- 2 large eggs
- Freshly ground black pepper, to taste
- ½ cup prepared salsa
- ½ medium avocado, sliced

Heat oil in a medium skillet over medium heat. Add the garlic, bell pepper, onion, and jalapeño pepper, and sauté until soft. Add the eggs and cook until the whites are cooked through. Season with freshly ground black pepper.

To serve, top the eggs and veggies with salsa and avocado. Serve immediately.

Serves 1

Classic French Omelet

Some dishes need to be adapted to fit the Paleo lifestyle, but a French omelet is one that fits perfectly. Well, almost perfectly. Most French omelets have cheese in them. If you try it without, however, you may find it's just as enjoyable. It may take practice to get the perfect visual effect, but the results are so delicious that you won't mind the practice it takes to get there.

- 3 large eggs
- 1 tablespoon olive or coconut oil
- 2 tablespoons chopped fresh herbs of your choice
- Freshly ground black pepper, to taste
- 2 slices minimally processed ham

Beat eggs in a bowl and set aside. Heat a non-stick skillet over medium heat and add the oil.

Add eggs, followed by herbs. Season with freshly ground black pepper. Cook for 1 minute and add the ham to the center. Once the eggs begin to cook, fold both sides toward the center.

Slide onto a plate and serve with extra ham slices and herbs for garnish.

Serves 1

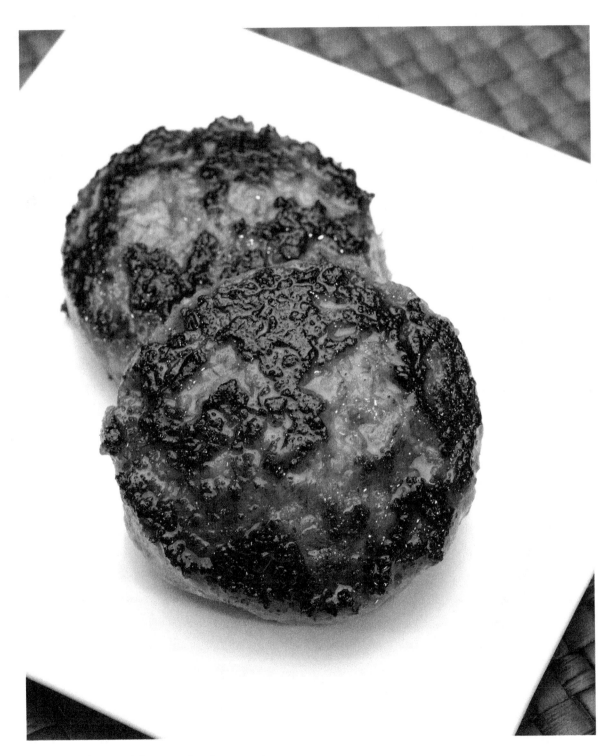

Homemade Breakfast Patties (page 24)

Homemade Breakfast Patties

While sausage technically fits on the Paleo diet, it can be hard to find a variety that isn't laced with added chemicals and fillers. Since you want to avoid these types of ingredients, making your own sausage is the best route to take. It's also one that is not nearly as difficult as it may sound, and the results are worth it. Feel free to adjust your seasonings to suit your personal tastes.

- 1 pound ground pork
- 1 teaspoon garlic powder
- 1 teaspoon paprika
- ½ teaspoon ground sage
- 1 teaspoon fennel seeds
- ¼ teaspoon cayenne pepper
- ¼ teaspoon white pepper
- 2 tablespoons olive or coconut oil
- Freshly ground black pepper, to taste

Using your hands, combine the pork with the seasonings in a large bowl until well combined.

Form into 8 to 10 patties. Heat a medium skillet over medium heat and add the oil. Fry the sausage patties until golden brown on both sides (about 4 minutes per side), making sure the inside is no longer pink. Season with freshly ground black pepper.

Serve immediately.

Serves 4

Paleo Western Omelet

Eggs are classics when it comes to Paleo diet recipes, and for good reason. High in protein as well as vitamins and minerals, they are what some would call a "super food." Even better, they are ridiculously easy to cook. This recipe has been modified just a bit to fit the Paleo diet, but you won't notice the difference, as it's super delicious.

- 3 large eggs
- 1 tablespoon olive oil
- 2 ounces minimally processed, thick-cut ham
- ¼ cup chopped bell pepper
- ¼ cup onion, chopped
- ½ cup spinach, finely chopped
- Freshly ground black pepper, to taste

Beat the eggs until frothy.

Add oil to a non-stick omelet pan and heat over medium heat. Add eggs. As they start to set, add the ham and veggies, spreading evenly throughout.

Fold over and finish cooking. Season with freshly ground black pepper. When eggs are thoroughly cooked, slide onto a plate and serve.

Serves 1

Caveman French Toast

While you might think the bread is the most important ingredient in French toast, you should try this recipe anyway. It's just eggs with French toast seasonings, and it really is quite delicious. Once you try it, it will probably become one of your favorite Paleo diet recipes. Make sure you use only real maple syrup, and not too much!

- 4 large eggs
- 1 tablespoon water
- 1 teaspoon vanilla extract
- 1 teaspoon cinnamon
- Pinch of nutmeg
- 1 tablespoon coconut oil
- Pure maple syrup for drizzling

In a small bowl, beat the eggs and water together until frothy. Add vanilla, cinnamon, and nutmeg.

Heat a non-stick omelet pan on medium-high heat. When hot, add coconut oil and swirl pan to coat.

Add half the egg mixture to the pan and let it cook through before flipping. Cook until browned on both sides.

Serves 2

Italian Frittata

Casseroles are comfort foods, and this one is no exception. A delicious recipe for a brunch, or even a lazy Sunday breakfast, this is one of the best Paleo recipes you'll find.

- 2 tablespoons olive oil
- 1 small onion, diced
- 2 cloves garlic, minced
- 1 zucchini, diced
- 1 pound spinach, coarsely chopped
- 12 cherry tomatoes, quartered
- ½ cup black olives
- Freshly ground black pepper, to taste
- 12 large eggs

Preheat oven to 375 degrees F.

In a large sauté pan, heat the oil over medium-high heat. Add the onions and garlic and cook until soft. Add the zucchini and continue cooking for a couple more minutes. Add spinach, combine and cook until wilted. Remove pan from heat and add the tomatoes and olives. Season with freshly ground black pepper.

In a large bowl, whisk the eggs until frothy.

Lightly brush the bottom of an 8 x 13-inch casserole dish with oil. Add the veggies to the dish. Pour over the egg mixture and stir to combine.

Bake for an hour until the top is browned and the center is cooked through. Slice into squares and serve.

Serves 6

Paleo Granola

Traditional granola doesn't work on the Paleo plan: It's loaded with oats, sugar, and other processed or high-carb ingredients. If you want something other than eggs for breakfast, this version fits the bill. It's got nuts, fruit, and coconut and is easy to prepare and store for a quick snack as well.

- 1 cup raw pecans
- 1 cup raw sunflower seeds
- 1 cup raw walnuts
- 1 cup raw sliced almonds
- 1 cup raw pumpkin seeds
- 1 cup unsweetened coconut, shredded
- 1 cup Medjool dates, chopped
- 1 cup raisins

Soak nuts and seeds overnight in warm water, about 10 hours. Drain well.

Spread the nuts and seeds on a baking sheet in an even layer. Set oven to the lowest temperature possible and put the baking sheet in the oven door open, dehydrate nuts for 10 hours. Allow to cool completely.

Chop nuts and seeds and combine with the coconut, dates, and raisins. Serve either as a snack or with unsweetened almond milk as a breakfast cereal.

Serves 8

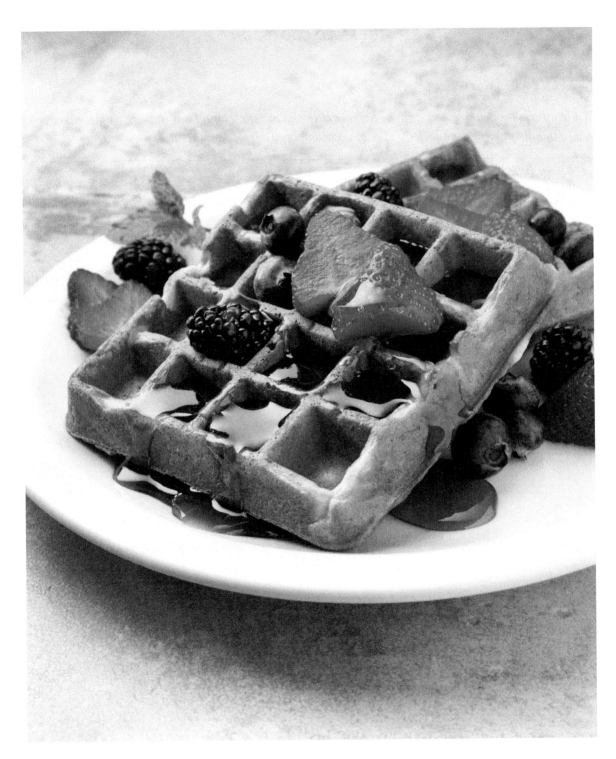

Paleo Waffles (page 30)

Paleo Waffles

While this isn't something you want to eat everyday, the use of coconut flour in these waffles allows you to indulge once in a while, for a special occasion, or just a weekend treat.

- ¼ cup coconut flour
- 4 large eggs
- 1 tablespoon coconut milk
- 1 tablespoon cinnamon
- ¼ teaspoon nutmeg
- ¼ teaspoon baking soda
- Pure maple syrup

Preheat a waffle iron. Blend all ingredients in a blender or by hand in a bowl. Pour batter in the center of the waffle iron, covering the entire surface area.

Cook until waffles release from the iron. Serve immediately with maple syrup.

Serves 2

Paleo Spinach Quiche

Traditional quiche is usually loaded with cheese, but you won't miss it in this flavorful recipe. It's a great dish to make the night before, especially if you already have the oven on for dinner.

- 1 teaspoon olive oil, plus more for greasing the pan
- 1 cup chopped fresh spinach
- ½ cup chopped red onion
- ½ teaspoon salt
- ½ teaspoon freshly ground black pepper
- ½ teaspoon ground nutmeg
- 8 large eggs, beaten
- ½ cup plain almond milk

Preheat oven to 350 degrees F. Grease a 9-inch glass pie plate.

In a small skillet, heat the olive oil over medium heat, and sauté the spinach, onion, salt, pepper, and nutmeg for about 5 minutes, or just until the onions are translucent.

Stir the eggs and almond milk together in a small bowl. Add the spinach mixture, stir, and pour into the pie plate.

Bake the quiche on the middle oven rack for 30 to 40 minutes, or until the center is completely set. Serve warm or at room temperature.

Serves 4 to 6

Banana-Berry Pancakes

These pancakes get their natural sweetness from berries and bananas. The recipe calls for raspberries, but you can substitute any type of berry. Berries are a great choice for the Paleo diet. They're high in antioxidants and add intense flavor and sweetness to any dish.

- 6 egg whites, lightly beaten
- 2 bananas, mashed
- ⅓ cup raspberries, mashed
- 2 tablespoons almond butter
- ¼ teaspoon cinnamon

Spray a skillet or griddle with cooking spray. In a large bowl, mix the egg whites, bananas, raspberries, and almond butter until smooth.

Pour the batter into the skillet using ½ cup for each pancake. Wait 2 to 3 minutes before flipping the pancakes. Cook an additional 2 to 3 minutes until golden brown. Serve with a sprinkling of cinnamon and/or fresh fruit.

Serves 2

High Fiber Bacon and Eggs

You probably don't think of fiber when you think of this classic high-protein breakfast, but the addition of shredded cabbage makes it just that. This is one breakfast that will fill you up and keep you full for hours, making it perfect for the busy day ahead of you. This makes a great quick lunch or dinner as well.

- 6 slices of uncured, nitrate-free, thick-cut bacon
- 1 tablespoon olive or coconut oil
- 2 cups cabbage, shredded
- Freshly ground black pepper, to taste
- 4 large eggs

Lay bacon on a sheet pan and preheat the broiler to high. Put bacon under the broiler and broil for 5 to 6 minutes per side, until desired crispness.

Heat the oil in a large skillet and add the cabbage. Cook until soft, browned, and lightly crisp. Season with pepper. Remove from pan and place on two plates.

Crack the eggs in the pan and cook until desired doneness. Season with freshly ground black pepper. To serve, place the eggs on top of the cabbage and serve with the broiled bacon.

Serves 2

Eggplant Holes

This is a Paleo take on the classic toast with a hole in it. Instead of bread, you use eggplant to get more nutrients, fewer carbs and, most importantly, an extremely delicious flavor. This is a dish you'll want to eat every morning for breakfast.

- 1 medium eggplant
- 2 tablespoons olive or coconut oil
- 4 large eggs
- Green onions, chopped, for garnish
- Freshly ground black pepper, to taste

Slice eggplant into 1-inch thick slices and season with pepper. Using a small cookie cutter, cut a hole in the center of each slice.

Heat a large skillet over medium-high heat. Add the oil, followed by the eggplant. Crack one egg into the center of each slice. Cook for 2 to 3 minutes and then flip, being careful not to let the egg fall out of the hole. Cook for another 2 minutes and remove from pan. Season with freshly ground black pepper. Garnish with the green onions and serve.

Serves 2

3

SANDWICHES AND WRAPS

Egg Salad Lettuce Wraps

When you first begin the Paleo diet, you'll find lunch is the most difficult meal to accommodate. It requires a bit of creativity, but you can still eat well—for example, with these lettuce wraps. Healthy, hearty, and delicious, this is sure to become a staple.

- 2 large hard-boiled eggs, peeled and chopped
- 2 tablespoons olive-oil mayonnaise
- 2 tablespoons relish or chopped pickles
- Freshly ground black pepper, to taste
- 2 large lettuce leaves, such as iceberg or romaine, intact and un-torn
- Lemon juice, for seasoning

Put chopped eggs, mayo, and relish in a bowl and mix thoroughly to combine. Season with freshly ground black pepper.

Divide the egg salad mixture evenly between the lettuce leaves and wrap, but not too tightly, as you don't want the leaves to tear. Season with lemon juice if desired.

Serve immediately with baby carrots for a healthy and filling lunch.

Serves 2

Sloppy Joe Cabbage Wraps

Using ground beef with a high amount of fat makes this dish a very filling choice. This recipe doesn't take long to prepare and is pretty satisfying. You might think the cabbage wraps don't fit, but with all the flavor from the Sloppy Joe mixture, you probably won't even miss the bun!

- 2 tablespoons olive oil
- ½ cup onion, diced
- ½ cup green bell pepper, diced
- 1 pound grass-fed ground beef
- Freshly ground black pepper, to taste
- 2 cups no-sugar tomato sauce
- 1 tablespoon chili powder
- Head of cabbage, leaves left intact and un-torn

In a large skillet, heat the oil over medium-high heat. Add onions and green bell peppers and sauté until soft.

Add ground beef and stir until browned. Season with freshly ground black pepper.

Add tomato sauce and chili powder. Simmer 5 minutes or until beef is cooked through.

To serve, spoon Sloppy Joe mixture into cabbage wraps, being careful not to overfill.

Serves 4 to 6

Chicken BLT

If you're looking for sandwiches while on the Paleo diet, most of the time you are going to be out of luck. That's okay because you don't need the bread, anyway. So what are you supposed to eat? Well, this pan-seared chicken breast with BLT fixings is a good substitute. Be sure to buy the best quality chicken you can find—and if you can get a good tomato, that just makes it better.

- 2 tablespoons olive oil
- 2 chicken breasts
- Freshly ground black pepper, to taste
- 4 large lettuce leaves, intact and un-torn
- Olive-oil mayonnaise, for serving
- Lemon juice, for seasoning
- 1 tomato, seeded and diced
- 4 slices uncured, nitrate-free, thick-cut bacon, crumbled

In a large skillet, heat oil on medium-high heat. Add chicken breasts and sear until browned. Flip over and finish cooking, making sure chicken is brown and crispy on both sides. Season with freshly ground black pepper.

When cool, slice chicken into strips.

Spread each lettuce leaf with mayo, being careful not to rip the lettuce. Add the chicken. Season with lemon juice if desired.

Top each with tomatoes and bacon and fold into wraps to serve.

Serves 2

High-Protein Grain-Free Burgers

This bun-less burger is kind of messy, and definitely something you're going to want to eat with a fork and knife, but you will be glad you did. Serve this with sweet potato fries if you wish, although the burger is filling enough alone. With burgers this delicious, it's a wonder there are people who still want to eat them with buns!

- 8 slices uncured, nitrate-free, thick-cut bacon
- 8 large eggs
- Freshly ground black pepper, to taste
- 1 pound grass-fed ground beef
- 1 teaspoon garlic powder
- 1 teaspoon onion powder

Heat a large skillet over medium-high heat. Add bacon slices, cook until crisp. Remove from pan.

Crack eggs and add them to the skillet individually, as many as will fit, and fry on both sides until cooked, seasoning with pepper. Remove from pan.

Season beef with garlic and onion powder and pepper. Divide into 4 patties. In a separate pan, fry each patty until cooked through.

To serve, place burger on one egg, top with two slices bacon, and top with another egg. Eat with a knife and fork for best results.

Serves 4

Chinese Chicken Lettuce Wraps

You'll find these tasty morsels on the menu of most swank Chinese restaurants, but ours have been adapted for a Paleo diet. Soy sauce is a fermented food, high in sodium and not particularly healthy. We've substituted garlic and tahini paste for flavor.

- 2 cups cooked chicken, shredded
- ½ cup green onions, sliced
- ½ cup carrots, shredded
- ½ cup slivered almonds
- ¼ cup cilantro, chopped
- Freshly ground black pepper, to taste
- 2 tablespoons olive oil
- 2 tablespoons sesame oil
- 2 tablespoons tahini paste
- ½ teaspoon ground ginger
- ½ teaspoon garlic, minced
- Lemon juice, for seasoning
- Bibb lettuce leaves, intact and un-torn

Combine the shredded chicken, onion, carrots, almonds, and cilantro in a mixing bowl. Season with freshly ground black pepper.

In a smaller bowl, mix the remaining ingredients to make a flavorful dressing.

Fold the dressing into the chicken mixture. Season with lemon juice if desired. Wrap the chicken mixture in lettuce leaves to serve.

Serves 4

Chicken Avocado Wraps

Avocado is high in fat, but it's the good, heart-healthy kind, so feel free to indulge. Choose avocados with firm skins that yield slightly to the touch. Store avocados at room temperature and allow them to ripen for up to one week. You can also peel avocados and store the flesh in the freezer to use later in guacamole.

- 2 cups cooked chicken, shredded
- ½ cup avocado, cubed
- ½ cup alfalfa sprouts
- ½ cup green onions, chopped
- ½ cup walnuts, chopped
- ½ cup basil leaves, chopped
- Freshly ground black pepper, to taste
- 2 tablespoons lemon juice
- ½ teaspoon dill
- 1 teaspoon honey
- 4 tablespoons olive oil
- Bibb lettuce leaves, intact and un-torn

Combine the chicken, avocado, alfalfa sprouts, green onions, walnuts, and basil leaves in a mixing bowl. Season with freshly ground black pepper.

In a smaller bowl, whisk the lemon juice, dill, and honey together. Slowly add the olive oil, whisking until it emulsifies and becomes thick and creamy.

Pour the lemon-dill dressing over the chicken mixture and toss to mix. Scoop the chicken mixture into lettuce leaves to serve.

Serves 4

SALADS AND DRESSINGS

Sweet and Savory Chicken Salad

A great combination of chicken mixed with fruits and vegetables makes this salad a unique and tasty treat. Unlike most chicken salads, the grouping of avocado and mayonnaise adds a flavorful side while the apples, grapes, and cranberries add a distinctly sweet side. Top with walnuts and celery to add an extra-crunchy texture.

- 4 boneless, skinless chicken breasts, cooked and shredded
- ½ cup dried cranberries
- 1 cup celery, chopped
- ¾ cup green grapes, halved
- ½ cup walnuts, chopped
- 1 avocado, peeled, pitted and diced
- 1 apple, peeled, cored and chopped
- 1 cup olive-oil mayonnaise
- Juice of 1 lemon
- Freshly ground black pepper, to taste

Combine the chicken, cranberries, celery, grapes, walnuts, avocado, and apple in a large bowl and mix well.

In a separate bowl, combine the mayonnaise with the lemon juice and whisk.

Add the dressing into the large bowl with the chicken mixture and toss until all are coated well in the dressing. Season with freshly ground black pepper. Serve chilled.

Serves 4

Conch Salad

Conch has a sweet, smoky flavor similar to clams. The conch is "cooked" seviche style in this dish by the acidity of the citrus. If you can't find conch at the market, scallops make a respectable stand-in. This is a great light lunch or dinner when you don't really feel like cooking a hot meal.

- 4 conch, cleaned with skin removed
- 1 small onion, chopped
- 1 stalk celery, chopped
- ½ small sweet pepper, diced
- 1 large tomato, sliced
- Juice of 2 limes
- Juice of 1 orange
- Freshly ground black pepper, to taste

Cut the conch into ¼-inch strips.

In a small bowl, toss the conch with all of the ingredients. Season with freshly ground black pepper.

Chill for 30 minutes before serving.

Serves 2

Tuna Salad with a Twist

Tuna is the perfect high-protein food for those following the Paleo diet. Green onions, jalapeños, ginger, and red chili flakes definitely give this salad a zesty bite. Served on a bed of lettuce, this dish makes for a satisfying meal.

- 2 cans white albacore tuna
- 1 cup green olives, chopped
- 2 green onions, chopped
- 1 jalapeño pepper, finely chopped
- 3 tablespoons capers, rinsed
- 1 tablespoon pickled ginger, chopped
- ½ teaspoon red chili flakes
- Juice of 1 lemon
- Juice of 1 lime
- 1 tablespoon olive oil
- 1 head butter lettuce or mixed greens
- 1 avocado, pitted and sliced
- Freshly ground black pepper, to taste

In a mixing bowl, combine all of the ingredients except the lettuce and avocado. Season with freshly ground black pepper.

Divide the lettuce between two chilled plates and place half the tuna mixture onto each. Arrange half of the avocado onto each salad and serve immediately.

Serves 2

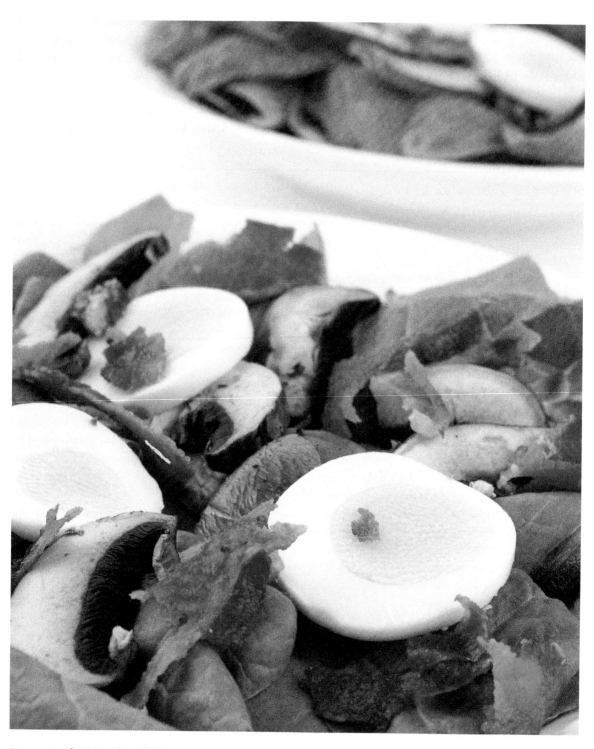

Bacon and Spinach Salad

Bacon and Spinach Salad

Bacon goes with everything but is especially nice with spinach. The walnuts and hard-boiled eggs add a nice variety of flavors and textures to this dish, making this a great salad for a full meal. You can also add a protein such as grilled chicken breast or a piece of broiled fish for a nice flavor profile.

- 1 pound fresh spinach, washed, drained, and torn into bite-sized pieces
- 1 can sliced water chestnuts, drained
- 1 pound fresh mushrooms, thinly sliced
- Freshly ground black pepper, to taste
- 6 slices uncured, nitrate-free bacon, cooked and crumbled
- ½ cup walnuts, chopped and toasted
- 4 large eggs, hard-boiled and sliced

Combine the spinach with the water chestnuts and mushrooms. Season with freshly ground black pepper. Divide between two plates.

Top with crumbled bacon, walnuts, and sliced eggs. Serve immediately.

Serves 2

Yam and Kale Salad

Yam and kale are both power foods loaded with essential vitamins and other good stuff that you need. The flavors of this dish are deep and satisfying, and this recipe can be a meal in and of itself. If you're looking for a little more, you can always pair this salad with roasted pork or even a tenderloin steak.

- 2 large yams, peeled and cut into 1-inch cubes
- 3 tablespoons olive oil, divided
- Freshly ground black pepper, to taste
- 1 medium onion, cut in half and sliced
- 3 cloves garlic, minced
- 1 pound kale, torn into pieces
- 2 tablespoons apple cider vinegar
- 1 teaspoon of thyme

Preheat oven to 400 degrees F.

Toss yams with 2 tablespoons of olive oil and season with pepper. Bake yams for 25 to 30 minutes or until tender. Allow to cool.

In a medium sauté pan, add the remaining tablespoon of olive oil. Add the onion and garlic and cook to a golden brown, about 3 minutes. Add the kale and cook for a few minutes until it wilts.

Combine the yams, kale, vinegar, and thyme together in a bowl. Season with freshly ground black pepper. Serve immediately.

Serves 2

Zucchini and Basil Salad

The flavors of this dish are very vibrant, like eating out of your garden. The hard-boiled eggs add a nice shot of protein for your diet, making this a great Paleo salad. It's filling, refreshing, and an excellent summer meal when you have way too many vegetables that you can't seem to put to use otherwise.

- 1 pound zucchini, shredded with skin on
- ½ cup fresh basil, chopped
- ¾ cup cherry tomatoes, halved
- 2 hard-boiled eggs, chopped
- 1 tablespoon olive oil
- 1 teaspoon thyme
- 1 teaspoon apple cider vinegar
- Freshly ground black pepper, to taste

Combine all ingredients and toss well. Season with freshly ground black pepper.

Serve immediately.

Serves 4

Brussels Sprouts and Beet Salad

Roasting the Brussels sprouts and beets really brings out the flavors of these satisfying vegetables. A touch of sweetness creates the perfect balance for the senses. If you are someone who thinks they don't like either of these somewhat controversial veggies, then you should try this salad. It just may change your mind!

- ½ pound Brussels sprouts, ends trimmed, outer leaves removed, cut in half lengthwise
- 4 tablespoons plus ⅓ cup olive oil, divided
- Freshly ground black pepper, to taste
- 4 small red beets, tops trimmed to ½ inch, washed, and cut in half lengthwise
- 1 tablespoon Dijon mustard
- 1 tablespoon honey
- Squeeze of lemon juice
- 1 small red onion, thinly sliced into rings

Preheat oven to 350 degrees F.

Toss the Brussels sprouts in two tablespoons of olive oil and place in a baking dish. Add pepper if desired, then roast until tender, about 20 minutes.

Toss the beets in two tablespoons of olive oil. Place beets onto a foil-covered cookie sheet. Roast in oven until tender.

Peel beets with a knife and cut into ¼-inch slices.

Make the dressing by whisking together ⅓ cup olive oil with mustard, honey, and lemon juice.

Toss the Brussels sprouts and beets with the dressing. Arrange the Brussels sprouts, beets, and sliced onion onto salad plates and serve warm.

Serves 4

Easy Greek Salad

Avocado, sun-dried tomatoes, and artichoke, along with crunchy onion and bell peppers, create a satisfying salad loaded with flavor—a nice variation on a classic Greek salad. For best results, use the freshest vegetables you can get your hands on.

- 2 tablespoons balsamic vinegar
- 3 tablespoons olive oil
- 1 teaspoon Greek seasoning
- 1 ripe avocado
- 1 green bell pepper, sliced
- ¼ medium red onion, sliced
- 1 cup black olives, pitted and cut in half
- 2 tomatoes, cut into bite-sized pieces
- ½ cucumber, halved and sliced
- ⅛ cup sun-dried tomatoes packed in olive oil
- ⅛ cup artichoke hearts
- Freshly ground black pepper, to taste

Whisk together the balsamic vinegar, olive oil, and Greek seasoning.

Combine the rest of the ingredients with the dressing. Season with freshly ground black pepper.

Let chill covered in the refrigerator for 30 minutes before serving.

Serves 2

Arugula, Prosciutto, and Cantaloupe Salad

Prosciutto is the perfect match to melon, bringing out the salty, savory flavor of the ham and the sweetness of the cantaloupe. The arugula adds a nice spicy contrast and the walnuts add a bit of crunch. This salad is best in the summer when you can get a fresh melon that is picked at the perfect time.

- 4 cups arugula, loosely packed
- 6 slices good quality prosciutto, cut into ½-inch strips
- ½ cantaloupe, seeds and rind removed, cut into ½-inch cubes
- 1 cup walnuts, roughly chopped
- Freshly ground black pepper, to taste
- Olive oil, to taste

Divide the arugula among four plates.

Top the arugula with prosciutto, cantaloupe, and walnuts. Season with freshly ground black pepper.

Drizzle a little olive oil over each salad.

Serves 4

Crab and Mango Salad

Crab is a good source of protein and omega-3 fatty acids. The mango adds a nice sweet-and-sour component to the salad. One bite of this salad and you'll think you're on an island in the Caribbean—especially if you can eat it outside on a nice sunny day.

- 4 cups mixed baby greens
- ¼ cup fresh cooked crabmeat, picked over for shells
- 1 mangos, peeled and diced
- ½ cucumber, peeled and sliced thin
- Juice from 2 limes
- 1 tablespoon fresh mint, roughly chopped
- 2 teaspoons olive oil
- Freshly ground black pepper, to taste

Divide the mixed lettuce between two plates.

Toss the remaining ingredients together in a bowl. Season with freshly ground black pepper.

Divide the crab salad between the two plates, heaping it in the center of the lettuce.

Serves 2

Shrimp with Mango Salad

Seafood is an essential ingredient in most any diet because it's so nutrient dense. This salad is a great introduction to seafood for those who have steered away from it in the past. The different flavors used in combination with the shrimp provide a very mild taste compared to other seafood dishes, such as mussels or oysters.

- 3 tablespoons fresh lime juice
- 2 tablespoons olive oil
- Freshly ground black pepper, to taste
- 2 large mangos, peeled, pitted, and diced
- 2 avocados, peeled, pitted, and diced
- 2/3 cup green onion, finely chopped
- 2/3 cup cilantro, finely chopped
- 1 pound shrimp, peeled and cooked

Prepare the vinaigrette by combining the lime juice with the olive oil in a small bowl. Season with freshly ground black pepper and set aside.

Mix the mangoes, avocado, green onion, cilantro, and shrimp in a large bowl.

Pour in the vinaigrette and mix well.

This salad is best served cold, so it is recommended that you keep it chilled if you are not serving it right away.

Serves 4

Mushroom Salad

This salad can be prepared with any type of mushroom. Portobello mushrooms will add a good meaty side to the taste, and they will also absorb the marinade, making them extremely flavorful. Wild mushrooms are another variety that will add a pleasant, yet distinct taste to your salad. Any fresh green may be used—arugula and baby spinach are two wonderful options.

- 2 tablespoons plus ¼ cup shallots, finely chopped, divided
- 3 tablespoons rice vinegar
- 11 tablespoons olive oil, divided
- 2 pounds mushrooms
- 1 teaspoon fresh thyme
- Freshly ground black pepper, to taste
- 6 ounces fresh greens

In a small bowl, combine the 2 tablespoons shallots and vinegar. Beat the mixture together and set aside for 5 minutes to permit the shallots to absorb the vinegar. Once they have absorbed the vinegar, mix in 7 tablespoons of olive oil and set aside.

In a large skillet over a medium-high heat, add the remaining oil. Add in the mushrooms and sprinkle with the thyme and some pepper. Depending on what type of mushrooms you use, the cooking time will vary. Add the ¼ cup shallots in with the mushrooms and continue cooking until the shallots are soft. Season with freshly ground black pepper.

Fill a large plate or bowl with the fresh greens. Place the mushrooms from the skillet on top of the greens and top with the vinaigrette.

Serves 4

Walnut and Beet Salad

Beets are a valuable root vegetable, low in saturated fat and cholesterol and a good source of dietary fiber and vitamin C. However, most people are not familiar enough with beets to use them regularly. This salad offers a quick and tasty way to incorporate beets into your diet.

- 4 medium-sized red beets, stems and ends removed
- ⅓ cup walnuts, chopped
- 2 tablespoons balsamic vinegar
- 2 tablespoons olive oil
- Freshly ground black pepper, to taste

Preheat oven to 400 degrees F. Wrap each beet in foil and place on a baking sheet. Roast in the oven for just about an hour.

Remove beets from the oven and allow to cool. Once cool enough to handle, remove them from the foil. While still warm, remove the skin of the beets. Plastic gloves are suggested so you do not stain your hands.

Slice beets into large chunks. Place in a medium bowl and mix in the remaining ingredients. Season with freshly ground black pepper. Allow beets to saturate in the dressing prior to serving.

Serves 4

Sweet-and-Sour Sweet Potato Salad

Combining a unique combination of flavors—from the sweetness of the apples and sourness of the lemon juice to the saltiness of bacon—this salad is a great complement to any barbeque and will be the talk of the town at your next potluck dinner. The potatoes and eggs offer a soft consistency, while the apples add a nice crunchy surprise to create a great balance of texture.

- 3 medium sweet potatoes, peeled and cubed
- Water, to cover potatoes
- 5 strips of uncured, nitrate-free bacon, roughly chopped
- 4 tablespoons olive oil
- 4 tablespoons olive-oil mayonnaise
- 2 tablespoons fresh lemon juice
- 1 tablespoon chopped chives
- 1 tablespoon Dijon mustard
- Freshly ground black pepper, to taste
- 3 hard-boiled eggs, chopped
- 1 green apple, chopped with skin still on

Combine the sweet potato cubes with water in a large saucepan over medium heat and bring to a boil. Cook until tender.

In a small skillet, fry bacon until crispy. Set aside.

In a small bowl, combine the olive oil, mayonnaise, lemon juice, chives, and mustard to create the dressing. Add fresh pepper as desired.

In a large bowl, combine the potatoes, eggs, bacon, and apples, then top with the dressing.

Serves 4 to 6

Spicy Scallop Salad

Scallops can be a terrific option, and they are quick and easy to make. They are an excellent source of vitamin B12, zinc, magnesium, selenium, and phosphorus, which many people lack in their diet. The cayenne pepper adds a little zing, and the scallops blend very well with it.

- 2 big handfuls of mixed greens
- 1 red bell pepper, seeded and cut into strips
- 1 avocado, cubed
- Juice of 1 lemon
- 1 teaspoon Dijon mustard

- 1 clove garlic, minced
- 2 teaspoons cayenne pepper
- Freshly ground black pepper, to taste
- ½ cup plus 3 tablespoons olive oil, divided
- 1 pound small sea or bay scallops

Combine the mixed greens, peppers, and avocado into a large bowl. Set aside.

Prepare the vinaigrette by stirring together the lemon juice, mustard, garlic, cayenne, and black pepper. Once combined, gradually mix in the ½ cup olive oil.

Rinse the scallops and delicately pat dry.

Heat a skillet over medium heat and add the 3 tablespoons oil and the scallops. Cook for approximately 2 minutes on each side until they are an opaque white color and just cooked through.

Combine the scallops with the bowl of mixed greens and veggies, and top with dressing. This is best served when the scallops are still warm.

Serves 4

Hot Chicken and Zucchini Salad

This is a hot salad featuring the unique combination of chicken and zucchini that is simple to prepare. Top with fresh almonds to complement the lemon and garlic mayonnaise.

- 2 pounds chicken breasts, cut into cubes
- 3 tablespoons coconut oil
- 1 large onion, chopped
- 5 zucchinis, cut into cubes
- 1 tablespoon dried oregano
- Freshly ground black pepper, to taste
- 7 tablespoons olive-oil mayonnaise
- Juice of 2 lemons
- 2 cloves garlic, minced very finely
- 1 head romaine lettuce, washed and shredded
- Sliced almonds, optional

Add the chicken cubes and coconut oil in a large pan over a medium-high heat until thoroughly cooked. Set aside.

Add the onion in the same pan and cook until soft, approximately 5 minutes.

Put in the zucchini cubes and oregano, and season with pepper. Cook until the zucchini cubes are soft.

Mix the mayonnaise, lemon juice, and garlic into a small bowl.

Add the cooked chicken, onion, and zucchini to the mayonnaise and stir well.

Add romaine lettuce, mix well, and serve in bowls. This hot salad is delicious topped with some almonds.

Serves 4

Canned Salmon Salad

Just because something comes from a can doesn't mean it can't be delicious. Salmon can be hard to come across, and even harder to keep fresh. Wild canned salmon can be a great addition to salad and is readily available as a cheap source year round. This recipe offers a complete meal with a distinctive taste and is very simple to prepare.

- 2 cans wild salmon
- Juice of 2 lemons
- 5 to 6 tablespoons olive oil
- 2 diced cucumbers, peeled or not
- 1 onion, chopped
- 1 large tomato, diced

- 1 avocado, pitted and diced
- 2 tablespoon fresh dill, chopped, optional
- Lettuce leaves for serving
- Freshly ground black pepper, to taste

Drain the liquid from the canned salmon, place in a bowl, and squash well with a fork.

Mix the lemon juice and olive oil into the salmon. Next, add the cucumbers, onions, tomato, and avocado and mix again. Add dill if desired. Season with freshly ground black pepper. Serve over cold lettuce leaves.

Serves 2

Pumpkin Salad

When you are looking for a simple and light salad for autumn, this is a great choice. If you are not a big fan of pumpkin, you can also substitute butternut squash instead. Roasting the pumpkin prior to making this salad will add a sweet flavor that is a great contrast to the arugula.

- 2 tablespoons olive or coconut oil
- 5 cups of pumpkin flesh or butternut squash, cut into ½-inch cubes
- Freshly ground black pepper, to taste
- 2 tablespoons orange juice
- 1½ tablespoons walnut oil
- Juice of 1 lemon
- ½ cup toasted walnuts
- 1 pound fresh baby arugula
- ½ cup fresh berries

Preheat oven to 450 degrees F.

Add the oil to a large bowl and mix with the pumpkin or butternut squash cubes. Add pepper.

Spread cubes on a baking sheet and roast for approximately 15 minutes. Turn the cubes over and roast for another 15 minutes until they are soft. Allow to cool at room temperature.

Mix the orange juice, walnut oil, and lemon juice in a bowl. Add the walnuts and arugula and stir to coat with the vinaigrette. Add pepper.

Add the roasted pumpkin or squash with berries and toss lightly.

Serves 6

Chicken Salad with Grapes

Shredded chicken is a staple of the Paleo diet. Full of protein, flavorful, and easy to prepare, keep some on hand at all times. One easy way to cook chicken in quantity is to cook 4 to 5 boneless, skinless chicken breasts in a slow cooker with a small amount of liquid. Shred the chicken and refrigerate it for quick Paleo meals. This chicken salad is just one of the many uses for shredded chicken.

- 2 cups cooked chicken, shredded
- ½ cup green onions, chopped
- ½ cup seedless grapes, halved
- ½ cup celery, chopped
- ½ cup almonds, slivered
- 2 large eggs

- 2 tablespoons lemon juice
- 2 teaspoons dry mustard
- ½ teaspoon cardamom
- 1½ cups grapeseed oil
- Freshly ground black pepper, to taste
- 4 cups mixed greens

Combine the shredded chicken, green onions, grapes, celery, and almonds in a large mixing bowl.

In a blender, mix the eggs, lemon juice, and seasonings. Slowly add the oil in a steady stream, blending until the mixture thickens and emulsifies.

Fold the homemade mayonnaise into the shredded chicken mixture. Season with freshly ground black pepper.

Serve on a bed of greens.

Serves 4

Southwestern Shredded Chicken Salad

You might find a lot of salads when searching out Paleo diet recipes, especially if you're looking for lunchtime meals. You'll notice that these are loaded with protein and veggies instead of the usual croutons and cheese, resulting in a satisfying take on what some might consider rabbit food. You'll also see that, instead of a creamy dressing, this salad is just topped with salsa—but don't worry, it's still delicious.

- 2 cooked chicken breasts, shredded
- 1 cup salsa, divided
- ¼ cup olive-oil mayonnaise
- 6 cups chopped iceberg and romaine lettuce
- ¼ cup black olives, sliced
- 1 small red onion, thinly sliced
- 1 avocado, pitted and sliced
- Freshly ground black pepper, to taste

In a medium bowl, mix the shredded chicken with ½ cup salsa and the mayo until thoroughly combined.

Divide the lettuce between two plates or bowls. Top each with half the chicken mixture, half the olives, onion, and avocado. Season with freshly ground black pepper.

Top each with half the remaining salsa and serve immediately.

Serves 2

Crunchy High-Protein Spinach Salad

Easy to put together, this salad travels well. Simply drizzle lemon juice over your apples to keep them from browning, and hold off on dressing the salad until right before serving. If this doesn't prove that Paleo diet recipes can be easy and quick, nothing will. Use any variety of apples you have, or even use two different ones for a flavorful twist.

- 6 cups tightly packed baby spinach
- 2 apples of your choice, cored and chopped, skin left on
- ½ cup chopped walnuts, toasted
- Freshly ground black pepper, to taste
- Olive oil and red wine vinegar, for drizzling

Divide the spinach between two plates or bowls.

Top with the chopped apples and walnuts. Season with freshly ground black pepper. Drizzle with oil and vinegar and serve immediately.

Serves 2

Chicken Fajita Salad

Who doesn't love fajitas? Unfortunately, they don't quite fit in with the Paleo diet as the basic components include flour tortillas and lots of sour cream and cheese. That doesn't mean you can't satisfy your cravings for fajitas though—it just means you need to be a bit creative.

- 2 boneless, skinless, chicken breasts
- Freshly ground black pepper, to taste
- 1 tablespoon olive oil
- 1 onion, sliced
- 1 red bell pepper, sliced
- 1 green bell pepper, sliced
- 1 yellow bell pepper, sliced
- 1 teaspoon chili powder
- 2 tablespoons lime juice
- 1 tomato, seeded and quartered
- ½ head each iceberg and romaine lettuce
- 1 avocado, pitted and sliced
- 1 cup prepared salsa

Heat a grill on high heat. Season with pepper and grill the chicken breasts until thoroughly cooked on the inside and nicely charred on the outside. Place on a cutting board and let cool.

In a large, heavy skillet, heat the oil on medium-high heat. Add the onions and peppers and cook until softened. Add chili powder and lime juice and let simmer until the liquid has evaporated. Add the tomato.

When chicken is cooled, slice.

To assemble the salad, divide the lettuce onto two plates, add half the pepper mixture and half the chicken. Season with freshly ground black pepper. Top with avocado slices and salsa and serve at desired temperature.

Serves 2

Everything Chicken Salad

This salad is a great Paleo recipe that contains a variety of ingredients for a flavorful meal. Think high protein and lots of veggies, and you're good to go.

- 2 boneless, skinless chicken breasts, cooked and cubed
- 3 large hard-boiled eggs, peeled and diced
- ½ head each iceberg and romaine lettuce, chopped
- ½ cup black olives
- ¼ cup olive-oil mayonnaise
- ½ cucumber, diced
- 1 tomato, seeded and chopped
- ½ cup sunflower seeds
- Freshly ground black pepper, to taste

In a large bowl, combine all of the ingredients.

Put in the fridge and chill for 30 minutes. Serve with a small fruit salad for a complete meal.

Serves 2

Bright and Sunny Chicken Salad

Tired of plain old chicken salad? This version really ups the volume with a curry mayonnaise and tropical fruit. Commercial mayonnaise is full of sodium and preservatives, but on the Paleo diet, you'll learn to whip up homemade mayonnaise in less than 2 minutes for a healthy and flavorful alternative.

- 2 cups cooked chicken, shredded
- ½ cup green onion, chopped
- ½ cup celery, chopped
- ½ cup grapes, sliced
- ½ cup mango, cubed
- ½ cup fresh pineapple, cubed
- 2 large eggs
- 2 teaspoons dry mustard
- 1 teaspoon curry powder
- 2 tablespoons lemon juice
- 1½ cups grapeseed oil
- Freshly ground black pepper, to taste
- 4 cups lettuce

Combine the shredded chicken, vegetables, and fruit in a large mixing bowl.

In a blender, mix the eggs, dry mustard, curry powder, and lemon juice. Slowly add the oil in a steady stream, blending until it emulsifies and forms a thick mayonnaise. Season with freshly ground black pepper.

Fold the curry mayonnaise into the chicken salad and serve on a bed of lettuce.

Serves 4

Salmon Salad

Heart-healthy salmon provides a hefty helping of omega-3 fatty acids for good brain and eye health. Use leftover grilled salmon in this tasty lunch salad.

- 1 cup cooked, flaked salmon
- ½ cup green onions, chopped
- ½ cup macadamia nuts, chopped
- ½ cup dried cranberries
- 4 cups mixed baby greens
- Freshly ground black pepper, to taste

- 2 tablespoons tahini paste
- 2 tablespoons sesame oil
- 2 tablespoons olive oil
- 1 teaspoon garlic, minced
- ½ teaspoon thyme

Combine the salmon, onions, nuts, cranberries, and baby greens in a large salad bowl. Season with freshly ground black pepper.

In a smaller bowl, whisk the remaining ingredients together to make an Asian-inspired dressing. Toss the dressing with the salad and serve immediately.

Serves 4

Tomato-Basil Salad

Visit a farmer's market and you'll find hundreds of varieties of tomatoes in a rainbow of hues. Most of these tomatoes are heirloom varieties and are far more flavorful than grocery store varieties, which are bred for long storage. Use a combination of tomatoes in this salad.

- 4 large tomatoes, cut in wedges
- ½ cup red onion, cut in rings
- ¼ cup packed basil leaves
- ¼ cup red wine vinegar
- 1 teaspoon garlic, minced
- ½ teaspoon thyme
- Freshly ground black pepper, to taste
- ½ cup olive oil

Toss the tomatoes, onions, and basil leaves together in a salad bowl.

In a small bowl, mix the red wine vinegar, garlic, thyme, and black pepper. Slowly whisk in the olive oil, until it is thick and emulsified.

Toss the dressing with the salad to serve. Season with freshly ground black pepper.

Serves 4

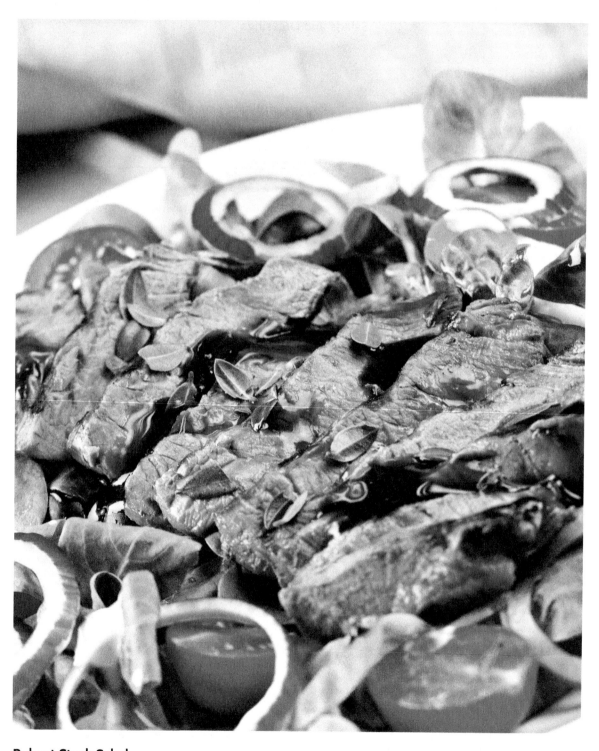

Robust Steak Salad

Robust Steak Salad

If you've limited your consumption of red meat in the past, rejoice! Red meat is allowed, and even encouraged on the Paleo diet. Seek out grass-fed beef from a reputable butcher. Grass-fed beef is higher in protein and lower in saturated fats than conventionally grown beef.

- 1 cup grass-fed steak, grilled and cut in thin slices
- ½ cup red onion, sliced in rings
- ½ cup cherry or grape tomatoes
- 4 cups baby greens
- Freshly ground black pepper, to taste
- ¼ cup red wine vinegar
- ½ teaspoon thyme
- 1 teaspoon dry mustard
- 1 teaspoon garlic, minced
- ½ cup olive oil

Combine the steak and vegetables in a salad bowl. Season with freshly ground black pepper.

Whisk the vinegar, spices, and garlic together in a smaller bowl. Add the olive oil in a slow drizzle, whisking until it becomes thick. Toss the dressing with the salad and serve immediately.

Serves 4

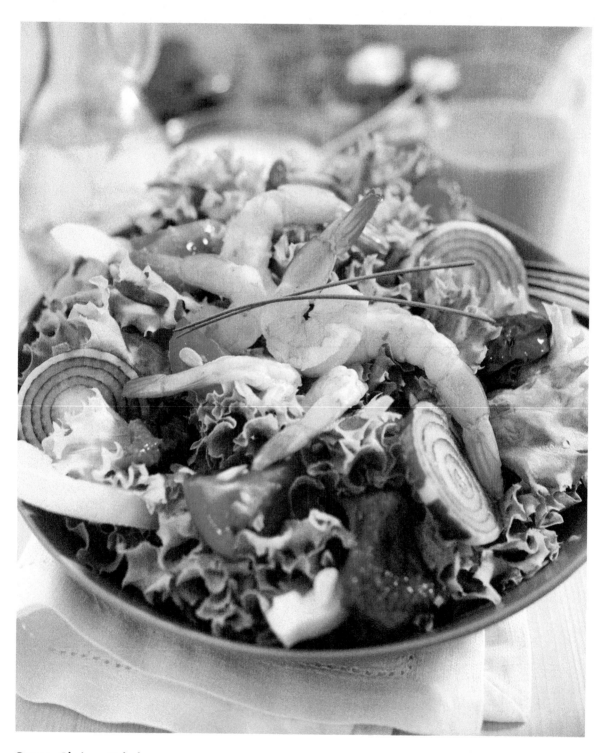

Savory Shrimp Salad

Savory Shrimp Salad

Shrimp, with its gently curving shape and delicate pink color, looks beautiful in salads and main dishes. It also pairs beautifully with bacon and avocado. Shrimp comes frozen in large bags labeled by the number of shrimp in each bag. The lower the number, the larger the shrimp. For this recipe, look for shrimp that has already been deveined and shelled.

- 1 cup shrimp, grilled or steamed
- 1 cup avocado, cubed
- ½ cup red onion, diced
- 2 strips of uncured, nitrate-free bacon, cooked and crumbled
- 4 cups baby greens
- ¼ cup fresh orange juice
- 1 teaspoon honey
- 1 teaspoon garlic, minced
- 1 teaspoon ginger powder
- Freshly ground black pepper, to taste
- ½ cup grapeseed oil

Combine the shrimp, avocado, red onions, bacon, and baby greens in a salad bowl.

In a smaller bowl, whisk the orange juice, honey, garlic, ginger powder, and black pepper. Slowly add the oil, whisking vigorously until it emulsifies.

Toss the dressing with the salad and serve immediately.

Serves 4

Sweet Broccoli Salad

Broccoli belongs to the cruciferous vegetable family and is related to cauliflower and Brussels sprouts. It has a mild, fresh flavor that pairs well with bacon in this salad to make a hearty lunchtime meal. Choose broccoli with closed buds, which are actually the flowers of the plant. Once the buds begin to open, the broccoli turns bitter.

- 2 cups broccoli florets
- 2 slices uncured, nitrate-free bacon, cooked and crumbled
- ½ cup red onion, chopped
- ½ cup grapes, halved
- ½ cup raisins
- ½ cup pecans, chopped
- Freshly ground black pepper, to taste
- 2 large eggs
- 2 tablespoons red wine vinegar
- 2 tablespoons dry mustard
- 2 tablespoons honey
- 1¼ cups grapeseed oil

Combine the broccoli, bacon, onions, grapes, raisins, and pecans in a mixing bowl. Season with freshly ground black pepper.

Blend the eggs, vinegar, mustard, honey, and black pepper in a blender. Slowly add the oil and blend until it emulsifies and becomes thick. Pour it over the salad and stir to mix. Refrigerate for at least 2 hours before serving for best flavor.

Serves 4

Spicy Tuna Salad

Think tuna salad is only for kids? Think again. This grown-up version combines chilies, peppers, and a chipotle mayonnaise for some kick. Natural tuna, canned in water, is high in protein and omega-3 fatty acids, making it a great value for the Paleo dieter.

- 2 cans water-packed tuna
- ¼ cup onion, finely minced
- ¼ cup red bell pepper, finely chopped
- ⅛ cup jalapeño pepper, finely minced
- 2 large eggs
- 2 tablespoons lemon juice
- 2 tablespoons dry mustard powder
- 1 teaspoon garlic, minced
- Freshly ground black pepper, to taste
- 2 tablespoons canned chipotle peppers
- 1½ cups grapeseed oil
- 4 cups lettuce

Combine tuna, onions, and peppers in a mixing bowl.

Blend the eggs, lemon juice, mustard, garlic, black pepper, and chipotle peppers together in another bowl. Slowly add the grapeseed oil, a few drops at a time, blending until thick and emulsified. Season with freshly ground black pepper.

Fold the mayonnaise into the tuna and serve on a bed of lettuce.

Serves 4

Tart Apple Coleslaw

This is a great side dish to bring to cookouts and is refreshingly sweet and tart from the addition of apples. Granny Smiths are the best choice for flavor and texture, but any apple will do in a pinch. If you use a sweet apple, you can omit the honey.

- ½ head green or purple cabbage, or a combination, grated
- 1 Granny Smith apple, grated
- 1 stalk celery, chopped
- 1 medium green pepper, diced
- ¼ cup olive oil
- Juice of 1 lemon
- 2 tablespoons honey
- 1 teaspoon celery seed
- Freshly ground black pepper, to taste

Combine all the ingredients in a bowl and toss well to mix. Chill for an hour or more before serving.

Serves 4

Classic Vinaigrette

This vinaigrette is a great basic dressing for almost any salad. The easiest way to prepare it is to put all ingredients in a jar and shake. Store in the jar and then you can shake again when you're ready to use more.

- ½ cup olive oil
- 3 tablespoons red wine vinegar
- 1 teaspoon Dijon mustard
- 1 garlic clove, minced
- 1 teaspoon honey
- Freshly ground black pepper, to taste

Put all ingredients in a jar, close the lid and shake until emulsified. Alternately, you can put everything in a blender and blend. Use to dress any salad right before serving and store the remaining dressing in the refrigerator for up to 3 days.

Makes ½ cup

Honey-Lime Vinaigrette

This is a great dressing for any southwestern-style salad. It pairs beautifully with tomatoes and avocado, and is even delicious on melon or peaches. Store extra in the refrigerator.

- ½ cup olive oil
- Juice of 1 lime
- 1 teaspoon honey
- ¼ teaspoon ground cumin
- Pinch chili powder
- Freshly ground black pepper, to taste

Put all ingredients in a jar or container with a lid and shake until combined. Use to dress salad right before serving.

Makes ½ cup

Orange Balsamic Vinaigrette

This sweet and tangy dressing gets its citrusy flavor from the addition of freshly squeezed orange juice and zest. The addition of mustard adds a little zip but also helps keep it from separating. This vinaigrette pairs beautifully over a spinach salad with fresh berries and red onions.

- ½ cup olive oil
- 2 tablespoons balsamic vinaigrette
- Juice and zest of one large orange
- 1 clove garlic, minced
- 1 teaspoon Dijon mustard
- Freshly ground black pepper, to taste

Put all ingredients in a jar or closed container and shake vigorously until emulsified. Use to dress salad right before serving and store any remaining dressing in the refrigerator for up to 3 days.

Makes ½ cup

Lemon Vinaigrette

This light and lemony dressing makes an excellent choice for a simple green salad without too many flavors and textures. It works beautifully on salads that have a grilled protein such as chicken or salmon as well, and you can easily customize it by adding herbs of your choice.

- ½ cup olive oil
- Juice of 1 lemon
- 1 teaspoon Dijon mustard
- 1 small clove garlic, minced
- Freshly ground black pepper, to taste

Put all ingredients in a jar or other container with a lid and shake until emulsified. Use to dress salad immediately before serving and refrigerate any remaining dressing for up to 3 days.

Makes ½ cup

Tomato Vinaigrette

This is a quick and easy take on a classic French dressing. While this version is not nearly as sweet as the bottled kind, it has a fresh tomato flavor that shines when tossed with baby greens.

- ½ cup olive oil
- Juice of 1 lemon
- 2 tablespoons Worcestershire sauce
- 10 cherry tomatoes

- 1 clove garlic, minced
- 1 teaspoon honey
- Freshly ground black pepper, to taste

Put all ingredients in a blender or food processer and puree until smooth and creamy. Add a little water a few drops at a time to thin out, if necessary.

Makes 1 cup

Caesar Dressing

While you can't have croutons with a Paleo Caesar salad, if the dressing is flavorful enough, you don't really need them. This version fits the bill, and it's much healthier than most bottled dressings. This is delicious over a seared or grilled salmon fillet and some fresh and crisp romaine lettuce.

- ½ cup olive oil
- 2 tablespoons olive-oil mayonnaise
- 4 garlic cloves, minced
- Juice of 1 lemon
- 1 tablespoon Dijon mustard
- 1 tablespoon Worcestershire sauce
- 3 to 4 anchovy fillets if desired, minced
- Freshly ground black pepper, to taste

Combine all ingredients in a blender or food processor and blend until smooth and creamy. Toss romaine lettuce with the dressing, top with desired protein or vegetables, and serve.

Makes ½ cup

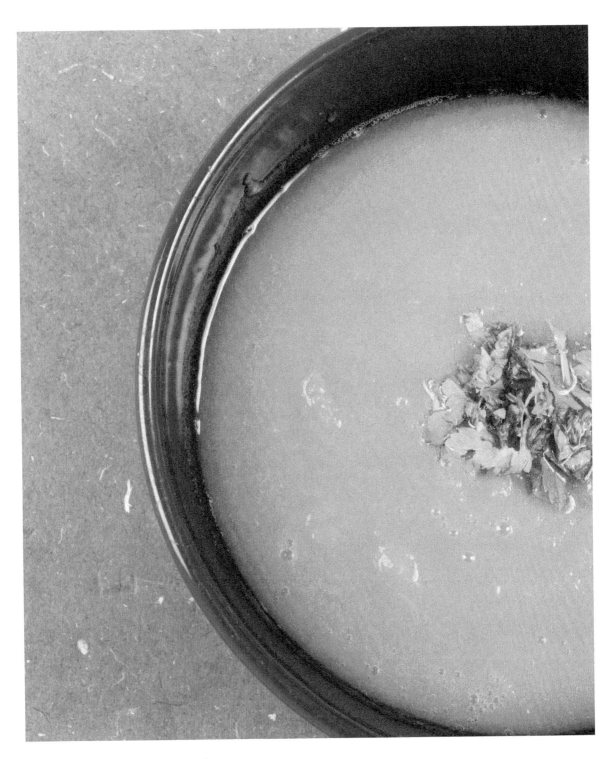

Classic Pumpkin Soup (page 82)

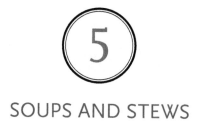

SOUPS AND STEWS

Classic Pumpkin Soup

Classic and simple, this recipe combines sweet potatoes and pumpkin to create a delicious and somewhat unusual soup. Don't let the simplicity of the ingredients fool you—it is bursting with flavor and makes a great soup for a lazy fall afternoon. Add a touch of cinnamon or nutmeg for a little extra spice.

- 2 tablespoons olive or coconut oil
- 1 onion, chopped
- 1 garlic minced
- 1½ pounds pumpkin flesh, chopped roughly
- 2 medium sweet potatoes, peeled and roughly chopped
- Freshly ground black pepper, to taste
- 4 cups chicken stock
- 1 cup canned coconut milk

Add the cooking oil to a large pot and simmer the onions in it until they are soft. Add garlic and simmer until you begin to smell the aroma.

Add chopped pumpkin and sweet potatoes, cook for a few minutes. Season with freshly ground black pepper.

Add the stock. Bring to a boil and let simmer for approximately 25 minutes, or until the sweet potatoes and pumpkin are tender.

Stir in the coconut milk.

Serve with an extra dash of coconut milk on top.

Serves 4

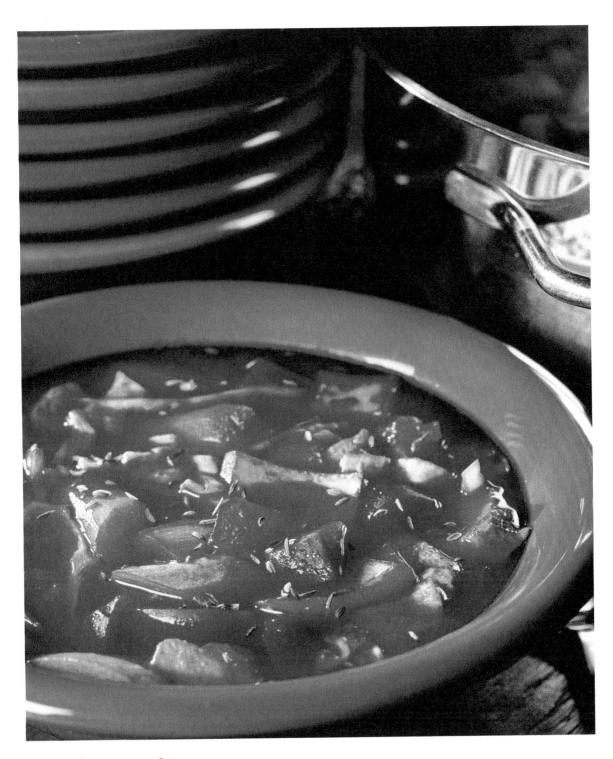

Beet-Red Soup (page 84)

Beet-Red Soup

This soup is a great idea around Halloween because of the vibrant red color that boasts a very close resemblance to blood. Extremely simple and easy to prepare, this would be a great soup for any Halloween party or cold October night.

- 3 tablespoons olive or coconut oil
- 1 medium onion, chopped
- 2 cloves garlic, minced
- 6 medium beets, scrubbed, peeled, and cubed
- 2 cups chicken broth
- Freshly ground black pepper, to taste

In a large pan, heat the oil and add the onion and garlic, stirring for approximately 5 minutes, or until soft. Add chopped beets and cook for another minute.

Stir in the chicken broth and season with fresh ground pepper. Bring to a boil and then reduce to a simmer for approximately 25 minutes, or until the beet cubes are tender.

Serves 4

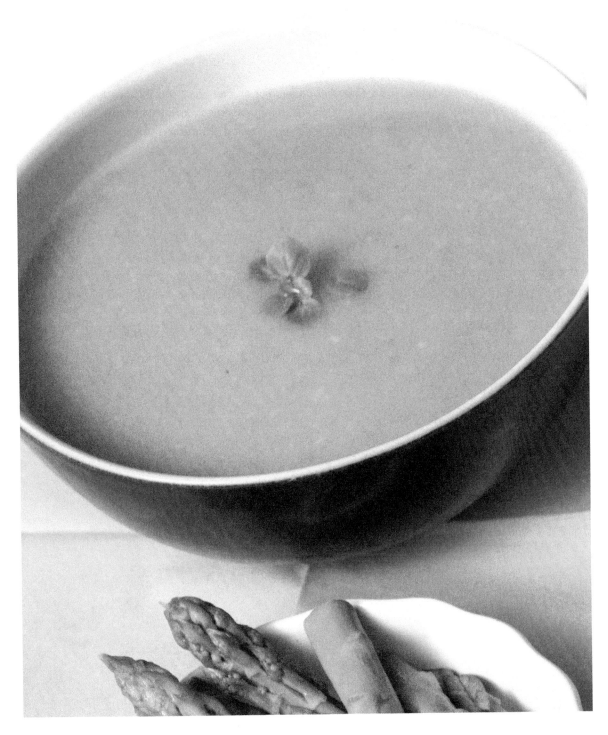

Cold Green Soup (page 86)

Cold Green Soup

This soup can be prepared using nothing more than a blender or food processor. The avocado adds a nice touch of richness to this otherwise quite light soup. The ingredients read like a list of health and nutrient-rich suggestions, and the ease of preparation will make this a welcome addition to your soup recipes.

- ½ pound asparagus, cut into 2-inch pieces
- 2 cups cold water
- ¼ pound spinach, stems removed
- 4 green onions, chopped
- 1 large cucumber, peeled and chopped
- 1 avocado, chopped
- 2 tablespoons lemon juice
- ¼ cup fresh mint leaves
- Freshly ground black pepper, to taste

Put the asparagus into a blender with ½ cup of the water and puree until smooth.

Add the spinach, green onions, cucumber, and another ½ cup of water. Blend again until smooth.

Add the avocado, lemon juice, and mint and repeat blending with the remaining water. Season to taste with pepper. Serve immediately.

Serves 4

Creamy Mushroom Stew

This stew is exceptionally filling as well as tasty. The coconut milk adds a good weight to the stew, and the portobello and white button mushrooms mixed with the oil add a taste that you won't soon forget. This can be served as a meal in itself or with a small side dish.

- 1 pound of portobello and white button mushrooms, stems removed and chopped
- 2 tablespoons olive or coconut oil
- 2 onions, chopped
- 4 cloves garlic, minced
- Freshly ground black pepper, to taste
- ¼ cup organic red wine
- ½ cup coconut milk
- Handful of fresh thyme, leaves picked
- 2 green onions, chopped

Rinse and pat dry all of the mushrooms.

Heat a sizeable skillet over medium heat. Heat the oil. Mix in the onions and garlic. Cook until they begin to brown, approximately 7 minutes.

Add in the mushrooms and season to taste with ground black pepper. After cooking for a few minutes, you will see that the mushrooms let off moisture. Continue to cook until this moisture evaporates completely.

Add the wine and the coconut milk and mix well to create an even distribution of flavor.

Let the stew simmer for a few minutes and then add in the thyme leaves and green onions. Allow to simmer on a low heat until it thickens. Serve immediately.

Serves 4

Creamy Asparagus Soup

Soups are surprisingly satisfying and are usually nutrient dense as well. Asparagus has a fresh, slightly acerbic taste that pairs well with the cream in this soup. Asparagus is available year-round, although it's at its best in the spring. Look for bright green stalks with closed tips. Open tips indicate the asparagus is old.

- 2 tablespoons olive or coconut oil
- ¼ cup finely chopped shallots
- 1 pound asparagus, steamed
- Freshly ground black pepper, to taste
- 2 cups chicken stock, preferably homemade
- 1 cup full-fat coconut milk
- 1 tablespoon organic white wine

Heat the oil in a large saucepan. Sauté the shallots for 5 minutes, or until tender. Place the shallots and the steamed asparagus in a blender or food processor and puree until smooth. Season with freshly ground black pepper.

Transfer the asparagus puree back to the saucepan. Add the remaining ingredients and heat to a simmer. Simmer for 20 minutes and serve.

Serves 4

Smoky Pumpkin Soup

Most pumpkin soups are somewhat sweet, but this one has a deep, smoky flavor and a bit of heat. Serve it on a cool, autumn day for an instant warm-up.

- 1 tablespoon olive or coconut oil
- ½ cup diced
- 2 strips uncured, nitrate-free bacon, diced
- 1 small can green chilies
- 1 cup pureed pumpkin
- 2 cups chicken broth
- ½ cup full-fat coconut milk
- ½ teaspoon chipotle chili powder
- Freshly ground black pepper, to taste

Heat the oil in a large saucepan. Add the onions and bacon and cook until tender, stirring frequently. Transfer the onions and bacon to a blender, along with the canned chilies. Puree until smooth.

Combine the pureed mixture with the remaining ingredients in the saucepan. Season with freshly ground black pepper. Heat to simmering, but do not boil.

Serve piping hot.

Serves 4

Chicken and Sweet Potato Soup

This delectable soup is a unique twist on chicken soup. With lots of herbs and spices and savory sweet potatoes, you'll love this healthy chicken stew.

- 2 tablespoons olive or coconut oil
- 1 small onion, chopped
- 2 cloves garlic, minced
- 1 medium carrot, finely diced
- 1 teaspoon thyme
- ½ teaspoon oregano
- 2 pounds boneless, skinless chicken thighs
- Freshly ground black pepper, to taste
- 4 cups homemade chicken broth
- 6 cups water
- 1 bay leaf
- 1 jalapeño, diced
- 1 large sweet potato, peeled and diced
- 1 bunch Swiss chard, leaves shredded and stems sliced
- 1 bunch green onions, chopped
- Juice of 1 lemon

Heat a large Dutch oven over medium-high heat. When hot, add oil, onion, garlic, carrot, thyme, and oregano, and cook until onion is softened and slightly translucent, about 8 minutes.

Cut chicken thighs into slices and season with pepper if desired. Add chicken to pot and continue to cook for another 10 minutes, stirring occasionally.

Reduce heat to medium, add chicken broth, 6 cups water, bay leaf, jalapeño, sweet potato, chard, and green onions and simmer for 20 minutes. Season with freshly ground black pepper.

Add the lemon juice and serve immediately.

Serves 6

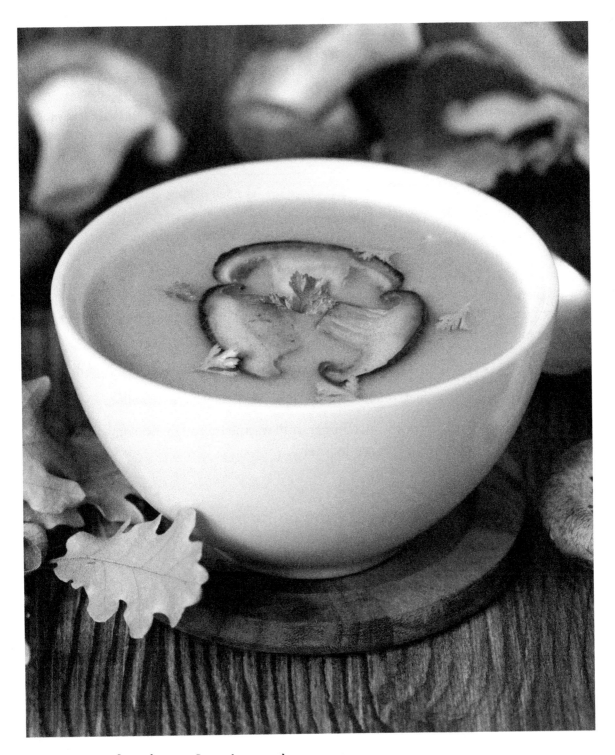

Paleo Cream of Mushroom Soup (page 92)

Paleo Cream of Mushroom Soup

This delicious creamed soup gets it's texture from avocado. It's a filling and flavorful soup that makes a great starter course to a Paleo dinner, but it can also make a light meal in itself when served with a green salad.

- 2 ripe avocados
- Juice of 1 lemon
- 2 cloves garlic, minced
- 2 cups water
- 1 tablespoon olive or coconut oil
- 1 mushroom, sliced
- 1 red bell pepper, diced
- ½ small onion, diced
- 2 tomatoes, seeded and diced
- Fresh chopped basil, for garnish
- Freshly ground black pepper, to taste

In a food processor, blend avocado, lemon juice, garlic, and 2 cups water. Set aside.

Meanwhile, heat a medium saucepan with tall sides over medium-high heat. Add the oil.

Sauté mushrooms, bell pepper, onion, and tomatoes until they begin to soften.

Add the blended avocado mixture and simmer until warmed through. Season with basil and freshly ground black pepper. Serve immediately.

Serves 4

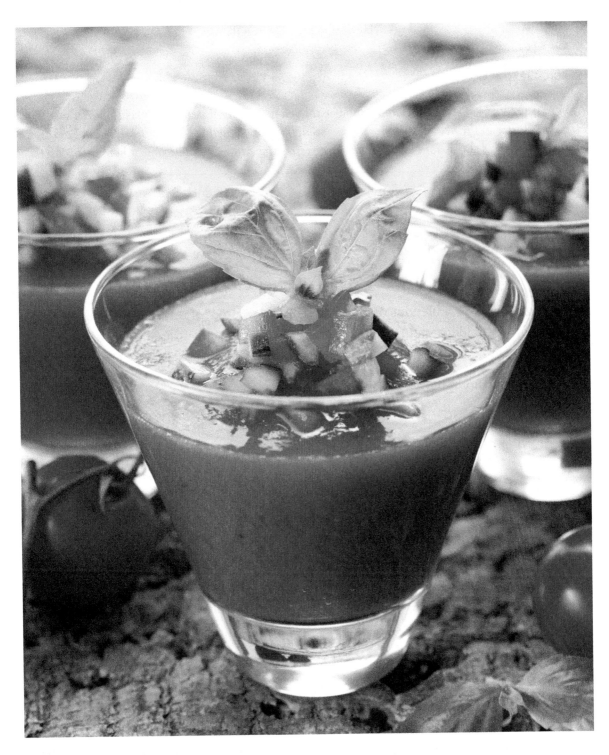

Classic Gazpacho (page 94)

Classic Gazpacho

If you've never had gazpacho, you don't know what you're missing. Essentially a cold soup, it's a refreshing starter in the heat of summer when you don't want something hot, but can't stand to eat another salad. This classic tomato version is easy, refreshing, and sure to become a household staple.

- 4 large, ripe tomatoes, roughly chopped
- 1 small onion, chopped
- 1 medium cucumber, peeled and chopped
- 1 small bunch fresh parsley
- 1 clove garlic, chopped
- Juice of 1 lemon
- 1 cup ice-cold water
- Freshly ground black pepper, to taste

Put all ingredients in a blender or food processor and process until vegetables are finely chopped. If you would like a pureed soup, continue blending until desired consistency. Season with freshly ground black pepper.

Chill for at least 1 hour and serve cold.

Serves 4

Vegetable Beef Soup

This is a classic beef vegetable soup with a few spices thrown in for added flavor. Feel free to use whatever vegetables you have on hand or whatever you like best to customize it to your tastes.

- 2 tablespoons olive or coconut oil
- 1 onion, diced
- 1 pound grass-fed beef stew meat
- 2 cups homemade beef stock
- 2 stalks celery, chopped
- 4 medium carrots, sliced into rounds
- 1 pound fresh baby spinach
- 1 tablespoon fresh parsley, chopped
- ½ teaspoon coriander
- ½ teaspoon garlic powder
- ¼ teaspoon ground marjoram
- Freshly ground black pepper, to taste
- Lemon juice, for seasoning

Heat a large Dutch oven over medium-high heat.

When pan is hot, add the oil and onion. Cook for 3 minutes until onions are lightly browned.

Add beef and brown for 5 to 6 minutes, stirring occasionally.

Turn heat down to medium-low, and add the rest of the ingredients to the pot. Season with freshly ground black pepper.

Simmer for 35 to 45 minutes, or until beef is tender and melt-in-your-mouth delicious. Season with lemon juice if desired. Serve immediately.

Serves 4 to 6

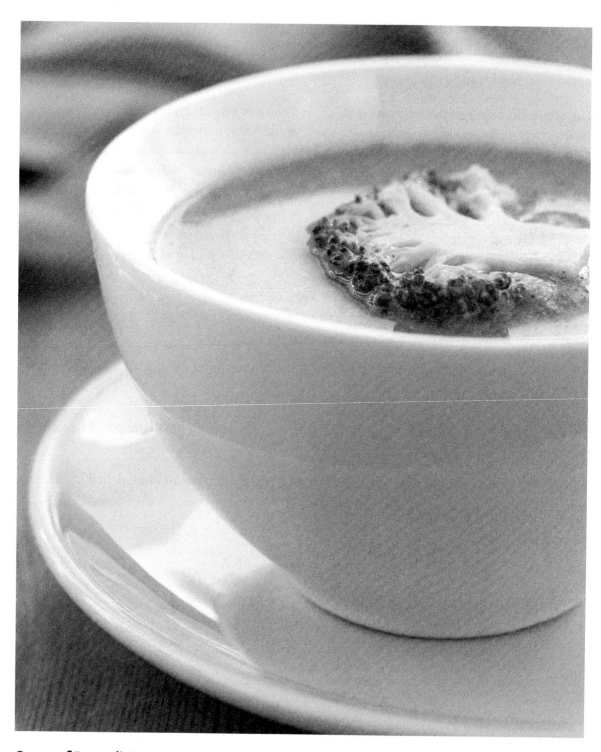

Cream of Broccoli Soup

Cream of Broccoli Soup

Cream soups traditionally rely on flour and cheese to thicken them, but pureed vegetables are really all you need. A bit of full-fat coconut milk adds a luxurious texture to this soup.

- 2 tablespoons olive or coconut oil
- ½ cup onion, chopped
- 2 cups broccoli, steamed
- 2 cups chicken stock, divided
- Freshly ground black pepper, to taste
- ½ cup full-fat coconut milk
- 1 teaspoon thyme
- ½ teaspoon nutmeg
- Lemon juice, for seasoning

Heat the oil in a skillet over medium heat. Add the onions and sauté them until they are tender.

Place the onions, broccoli, and ½ cup chicken stock in a blender. Puree until smooth. Season with freshly ground black pepper.

Transfer the broccoli puree to a large saucepan and add the remaining ingredients. Simmer for 20 minutes to heat through. Season with lemon juice if desired. Serve immediately.

Serves 4

Hearty Paleo Stew

Is there anything more satisfying than a big bowl of beef stew? This recipe is modified (although just slightly) to fit right in with the plan so you won't miss a beat. If you don't have turnips, you can just as easily substitute sweet potatoes.

- 4 slices uncured, nitrate-free bacon, diced
- 4 to 6 pounds grass-fed beef roast, cubed
- 1 small onion, finely chopped
- 2 garlic cloves, minced
- 2 large carrots, diced
- 2 turnips, diced
- 1 cup tomatoes, diced
- 1 teaspoon dried thyme
- Freshly ground black pepper, to taste
- 1 to 2 cups beef or chicken stock

Heat a large stockpot and add bacon. Cook until almost crisp, and add the cubed beef. Sear on all sides until golden brown.

Add onion and garlic, cook until both are soft, add carrots, turnips, tomatoes, and thyme. Simmer 5 minutes. Season with freshly ground black pepper.

Add stock and bring to a boil. Reduce heat and simmer 4 to 5 hours on low heat, or until beef is melt-in-your-mouth tender, and serve.

Serves 4 to 6

Spicy Southwestern Chicken Soup

Every culture has its version of chicken soup—all hearty and soul satisfying. And Grandma was right—chicken soup contains anti-inflammatory properties that can relieve cold symptoms, according to the University of Nebraska Medical Center. This chicken soup is perfect for the Paleo diet. It's chock-full of chicken (for protein) and tasty vegetables.

- 2 tablespoons olive or coconut oil
- ½ cup onion, chopped
- ½ cup red bell pepper, chopped
- ½ cup zucchini, chopped
- 1 teaspoon garlic, minced
- 1 (8-ounce) can roasted, chopped green chilies
- 1 (14-ounce) can diced tomatoes with chilies

- 4 cups chicken stock
- 2 cups cooked chicken, shredded
- 2 teaspoons cumin
- 2 teaspoons chili powder
- ½ teaspoon cayenne pepper
- Freshly ground black pepper, to taste

Heat the oil in a large stockpot. Add the onions, bell pepper, zucchini, and garlic and cook until tender.

Add the remaining ingredients and heat to simmering. Season with freshly ground black pepper. Simmer for 30 minutes and serve.

Serves 4

Not-Your-Grandma's Minestrone

Traditional minestrone includes beans and pasta, but this version is a hearty vegetable soup.

- 2 tablespoons olive or coconut oil
- 1 pound grass-fed beef stew meat
- ¼ cup onion, chopped
- ¼ cup celery, chopped
- 1 teaspoon garlic, minced
- 4 cups beef stock
- 1 (14-ounce) can diced tomatoes, with the juice
- 3 carrots, peeled and sliced in thin slices
- ¼ cup kale or spinach, chopped
- ¼ cup broccoli florets
- ½ cup zucchini rounds
- Freshly ground black pepper, to taste

Heat the oil in a stockpot over medium heat. Brown the stew meat and add the onions, celery, and garlic, cooking until the vegetables become tender.

Add the remaining ingredients to the stockpot and raise the heat to simmering. Simmer for 20 to 30 minutes. Season with freshly ground black pepper. Serve hot.

Serves 4

Veggie Soup with a Kick

While this is not a vegetarian recipe, it is loaded with filling, high-fiber vegetables and lots of protein. Fresh vegetables work well here, and you can substitute whatever you have or like—just be sure to stay away from starchy vegetables like white potatoes and corn.

- 4 slices uncured, nitrate-free, thick-cut bacon, diced
- 1 onion, diced
- 1 green bell pepper, diced
- 2 medium carrots, diced
- 2 zucchini, diced
- ½ head cabbage, shredded
- 1 pound grass-fed ground beef
- 1 cup canned tomatoes with juice
- 1 tablespoon chili powder
- ½ teaspoon cayenne pepper
- 2 cups chicken or beef stock
- Freshly ground black pepper, to taste

Heat a large pot or Dutch oven over medium-high heat. Add the bacon and cook until crisp.

Add the onion and bell pepper and cook until softened.

Add carrots, zucchini, and cabbage, cooking until carrots are slightly tender, approximately 5 minutes.

Add ground beef and cook until browned, and then add tomatoes and seasonings, followed by stock. Bring to a boil.

Reduce heat and simmer until carrots and beef are cooked through. Season with freshly ground black pepper. Serve piping hot.

Serves 6

I added more stock

Velvety Squash Soup

Apples and butternut squash complement each other perfectly and are widely available in the fall. Try roasting the two together for a dinner side dish, and save enough to make this tasty soup. Butternut squash stores well in a cool pantry, but you can also freeze cubed butternut squash for later use.

- 2 tablespoons olive or coconut oil
- 2 cups butternut squash, peeled and cubed
- 1 cup apples, peeled, cored, and quartered
- ½ cup shallots
- 4 cups chicken stock
- ½ cup full-fat coconut milk
- ½ teaspoon thyme
- Freshly ground black pepper, to taste
- 2 strips uncured, nitrate-free bacon, cooked and crumbled

Preheat oven to 450 degrees F. Heat the oil in the microwave. Spread the butternut squash, apples, and shallots on a baking sheet. Add the olive or coconut oil and toss to coat. Roast for 15 to 25 minutes, or until tender, stirring frequently so the shallots don't burn.

Transfer the squash, shallots, and apples to a blender or food processor and puree until smooth. Pour the mixture into a stockpot and add the stock, coconut milk, and thyme. Season with freshly ground black pepper. Simmer for 20 minutes. Top with crumbled bacon.

Serve piping hot.

Serves 6

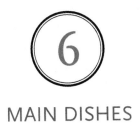

MAIN DISHES

Beef

Classic Diner Steak and Eggs

Two keystones of the Paleo diet, steak and eggs, make a classic combination that has been served for ages. This is a simple recipe that can be enjoyed in the morning for breakfast or in the evening for a quick dinner. The eggs can be prepared however you like, although traditional steak and eggs are prepared with sunny-side-up eggs.

- 2 tablespoons olive or coconut oil
- 1 grass-fed steak fillet of your choice
- Freshly ground black pepper, to taste
- 2 large eggs
- Paprika to taste

Heat a pan over a medium-high heat, and heat 1 tablespoon of the oil. Lightly season steak with freshly ground black pepper.

Cook the steak to your favorite temperature. Approximately 3 minutes on each side will usually give you a medium-rare steak.

Take out the steak, set aside, and lower the temperature to medium-low. Add the remaining oil.

Crack open the eggs in the hot pan, cover and cook them however you would like them prepared. Season with freshly ground black pepper and paprika. Serve with the steak immediately.

Serves 1

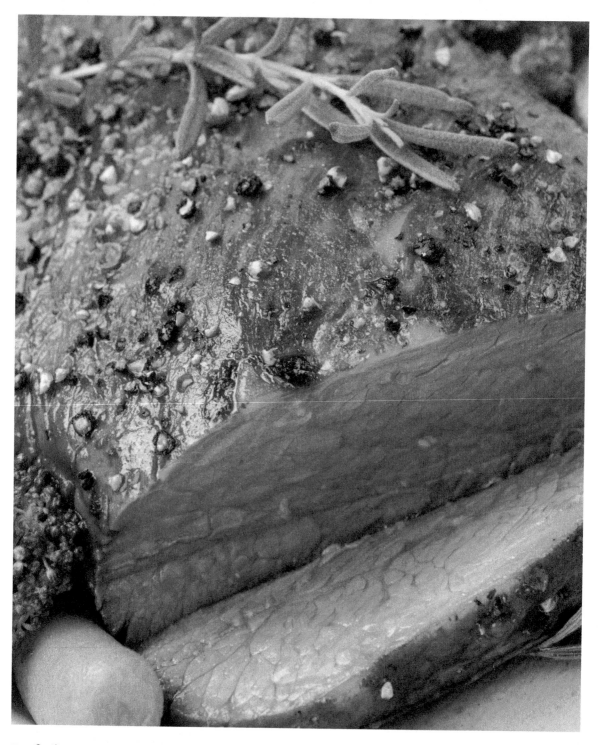

Beef Rib Roast with a Green Peppercorn Sauce

Beef Rib Roast with a Green Peppercorn Sauce

The next time you are in charge of cooking for guests, a prime beef rib roast is a delicious, juicy dish that will have them raving about the meal for years to come. This cooking method will create an amazing juice that is then used to create an unforgettable peppercorn sauce.

- 1 (6-pound) grass-fed beef rib roast
- 1 medium onion, chopped
- 3 garlic cloves, minced
- 1 medium carrot, sliced
- Pinch dried thyme
- 2 tablespoons olive or coconut oil plus additional as needed
- Freshly ground black pepper, to taste
- ½ cup organic red wine
- 1 cup beef stock
- 2 tablespoons green peppercorns

Preheat oven to 400 degrees F.

Trim some of the excess fat off the rib points and the roast itself. This fat will be used to help create the sauce.

Put the trimmed fat into a roasting pan and add the onion, garlic, carrot, and thyme.

Add a generous amount of olive or coconut oil. Place the pan in the oven and roast for approximately 20 minutes, or until golden.

Remove the pan from the oven, put the roast on top of the vegetables and fat parts, and season with pepper and some more thyme. Add more oil.

Place the pan with the roast back into the oven and roast for 45 minutes.

Lower the oven temperature to 350 degrees F and cook for another 45 minutes for a medium-rare roast.

Take the pan out of the oven and remove the roast. Set the roast aside, freely covered with a piece of parchment or aluminum foil, for approximately 15 minutes.

Place the roasting pan on the stovetop and deglaze it with red wine. Be sure to scrape the pan considerably with a wooden spoon. Boil and reduce the liquid to one-third. Add beef stock and boil for another 5 minutes.

Add the green peppercorns and squash them with a fork. Season with freshly ground black pepper.

Serve immediately with slices of rib roast.

Serves 8 to 10

Wrapped Roast Beef with Mustard and Horseradish

The process of roasting meat can be intimidating to some, but this very simple recipe has few directions and contains ingredients you probably already have on hand. A visit to your butcher for a select cut of fresh beef will make a great deal of difference in the end, and the combination of horseradish and mustard are superb.

- ¼ cup olive or coconut oil
- 3 cloves garlic, minced
- 1 tablespoon Dijon mustard
- 1 tablespoon horseradish
- Freshly ground black pepper, to taste

- 3½-pound grass-fed top sirloin roast beef
- 6 slices uncured, nitrate-free bacon
- ¾ cup organic red wine
- 1¾ cups beef stock

Preheat oven to 400 degrees F.

Mix the oil, garlic, mustard, and horseradish in a small bowl. Blend until smooth. Season with freshly ground black pepper.

Rub the roast completely with the mixture.

Arrange the bacon out flat so that the slices are somewhat overlapping. Place the roast on top of the bacon. Wrap the pieces around the roast. Use toothpicks to hold the bacon in place if needed.

Place the roast in a roasting dish and cook for 20 minutes. Add the wine and stock to the roasting dish and adjust the heat to 350 degrees F.

Roast for an hour, remove from oven, and allow to rest before serving.

Serves 4

Roast Beef with Thyme, Garlic, and Organic Red Wine

Although simple to prepare, this recipe does require a little cooking time, so make sure you start early. You should not take short cuts when it comes to purchasing the meat—top sirloin is used for the marbling fat that will add the main source of flavor, as well as provide a healthy source of energy.

- ½ cup olive or coconut oil, divided
- 4-pound grass-fed top sirloin roast
- 3 tablespoons Worcestershire sauce
- ¾ cup organic red wine
- 3 cloves garlic, minced
- Freshly ground black pepper, to taste
- 3 sprigs fresh thyme

Heat 1 tablespoon of the oil in a large skillet. Sear the roast on all sides for just a few moments, or until the sides are a beautiful golden brown.

Place the roast in a large roasting dish, along with the oil used to sear it. Add generous amounts of remaining oil on top of the roast, followed by the Worcestershire sauce and red wine. Sprinkle the garlic over the meat and season to taste with pepper. Top with the thyme sprigs.

Allow to cook for 50 to 60 minutes, or until the meat is just a little pink in the middle. Baste the meat with the cooking juices to keep it really moist.

Remove from the oven and set aside for approximately 10 minutes before serving, allowing the meat to cool before carving it.

Remove the thyme sprigs and use the liquid in the pan as a sauce.

Serves 4 to 5

Beanless Chili

A complete dish on its own, this chili doesn't need beans, which can be full of phytates and lections. Unlike most chili recipes, this is a very mild recipe and produces a thick and hearty result in the end. This chili is a quick stovetop meal that is simple to prepare and is great for a snowy winter afternoon in front of the fireplace.

- 5 pounds grass-fed ground beef
- 1 tablespoon olive oil plus additional add as needed
- 6 cloves garlic, minced
- 1 onion, finely chopped
- 5 celery stalks, chopped
- 5 carrots, chopped
- 4 cups button mushrooms, chopped
- Freshly ground black pepper, to taste
- 3 (28-ounce) cans crushed tomatoes
- 3 bay leaves
- 3 thyme sprigs
- 2 tablespoons fresh parsley, chopped

In a large skillet, cook the ground beef. Add oil if needed.

Sauté the garlic in olive oil in a very large saucepan over medium heat. Cook for approximately 2 minutes, or until the garlic is aromatic.

Add the onion, celery, carrots, and mushrooms, and stir well. Cook for another 5 to 10 minutes, or until the vegetables are soft. Season with freshly ground black pepper.

Add canned tomatoes, followed by cooked ground beef. Stir well. Drop in the bay leaves, thyme, and parsley.

Season to taste with pepper, reduce the heat to low, and simmer, uncovered, for about 4 hours, or until thick, stirring intermittently.

Serve immediately.

Serves 8

Hearty Mushroom Meatloaf

The ingredients holding this meatloaf together are not what you would expect in a meatloaf recipe. Eggs and mushrooms are the main ingredients, and when topped with honey, Worcestershire sauce, and ketchup, the combination creates a subtly sweet and salty taste.

- 1 tablespoon olive or coconut oil
- 2 cups white button mushrooms, finely chopped
- 2 pounds grass-fed ground beef
- 1 large egg
- 1 medium onion, finely chopped
- 1 teaspoon chili pepper flakes
- 3 teaspoons fresh thyme, minced
- 1 teaspoon fresh oregano, minced
- 3 cloves garlic, minced
- Freshly ground black pepper, to taste
- ½ cup ketchup
- 1 tablespoon honey, optional
- ½ tablespoon Worcestershire sauce, optional

Preheat oven to 350 degrees F.

Heat the oil in a medium-sized skillet, add the mushrooms and sauté for 2 to 3 minutes, or until the mushrooms are soft and browned.

Combine the meat, egg, onion, chili pepper, thyme, oregano, garlic, and pepper in a large bowl. Mix well. Add the cooked mushrooms as well, making sure they are evenly dispersed.

Place in a lightly greased loaf pan, and place in the oven to cook for approximately 15 minutes.

In a small bowl, combine ketchup, honey, and Worcestershire sauce. After cooking for 15 minutes, add sauce on the top of the loaf. Continue cooking for another 40 minutes before serving.

Serves 6

Herb- and Prosciutto-Stuffed Steak

Prosciutto is a dry-cured ham of Italian origin and is very thinly sliced. It's very salty, with a nice meaty taste. This recipe combines the flavors of the prosciutto, herbs, and vegetables to create one of the most flavorful steaks you will ever have. Stuffed steak is simpler to prepare than you would think, and the effort is well worth the reward.

- ¼ cup olive oil
- ¼ cup organic red wine
- 2 cloves garlic, minced
- Freshly ground black pepper, to taste
- 1 grass-fed flank steak or other thick steak
- 6 slices good quality prosciutto
- 1 red bell pepper, chopped
- 3 tablespoons fresh parsley, finely chopped
- 12 fresh basil leaves, finely chopped

In a bowl large enough to hold the steak, combine the olive oil, wine, garlic, and pepper. Mix together.

Butterfly the steak so that there is a seam along the middle.

Put the steak in the marinade and marinade for about 1 to 2 hours at room temperature.

Preheat oven to 350 degrees F.

Remove the steak from the marinade and keep the remaining marinade for later. Lay the steak open and stuff with prosciutto, bell pepper, 2 tablespoons parsley, and three-quarters of the basil. Season with freshly ground black pepper.

Have the steak vertically in front of you and roll firmly. You may need strings to keep the roll closed as it cooks.

Place on baking sheet, cover in remaining marinade, and sprinkle with remaining herbs.

Put in the preheated oven and let cook for 30 minutes. Allow to rest for 10 minutes before serving.

Serves 3

Portobello Burgers

Pretty much anything goes when you are topping these burgers. Make sure to use a ground beef that is lean, but not too lean. You want a little bit of fat in the meat to add more flavor. Using the portobello mushrooms as the bun offers a nice alternative to bread, as well as a unique taste. Add your favorite vegetables, just as you would with any burger. Avocados add a nice taste as well.

- 3 pounds grass-fed ground beef
- 3 large eggs
- 2 cloves garlic, minced
- Freshly ground black pepper, to taste
- 8 to 12 large portobello mushrooms
- 2 tablespoons olive oil

Place ground beef in a bowl and mix with the eggs. Add in the garlic and season lightly with pepper. Form 6 to 8 patties that are smaller than the mushroom caps.

Put on a preheated grill and cook each side for about 5 to 7 minutes. Rinse mushrooms and pat dry. Remove the mushroom stems.

Coat the caps in olive oil and then season with pepper. Do not let the oil penetrate for long to keep the mushrooms from getting soggy.

Place on preheated grill and cook on each side for about 5 to 7 minutes. Add hamburger patty and top as desired.

Serves 4 to 6

Citrus Beef Stir-Fry

Served on a bed of fresh citrus fruits, this beef recipe is a light combination of stir-fry and salad. The citrus juice offers a nice tangy taste to the beef, and the preparation is simple and offers a beautiful presentation that will impress your family and friends.

- 2 tablespoons olive or coconut oil plus additional as needed
- 1 pound grass-fed tender beef, cut into thin strips
- 1 onion, thinly sliced
- 2 garlic cloves, minced
- 1 teaspoon ginger, grated
- 1 tablespoon orange juice
- 1 tablespoon lemon juice
- 1 teaspoon lemon zest
- 1 teaspoon orange zest
- A big bunch of spinach
- Freshly ground black pepper, to taste
- 1 lemon, sliced
- 1 orange, sliced

Heat the oil in a large skillet or wok. Add the beef and stir-fry, turning constantly.

Remove the beef from the wok, then make sure the wok regains its temperature before you add more oil and stir-fry the onion, garlic, and ginger for approximately 3 minutes.

Place the beef back in the wok and then add the orange, lemon juice, and zest. Bring to a boil and add the spinach.

Cook until spinach is just wilted. Season with freshly ground black pepper.

Serve on a bed of citrus with the sliced lemon and orange.

Serves 2

Flintstone Rib Eye

The rib eye steak is one of the most extravagant steaks around—marbled with fat, and naturally juicy and tender. On the Paleo diet, you can enjoy steak, especially grass-fed steak, once a week or more. Although rib eye needs little more than a dusting of black pepper, this marinade adds extra flavor.

- ¼ cup olive oil
- 2 teaspoons garlic, minced
- 2 tablespoons tahini paste
- 2 grass-fed rib eye steaks
- Freshly ground black pepper, to taste

Mix the olive oil, garlic, and tahini paste in a bowl. Place the rib eye steaks in a shallow dish and cover them with the marinade. Lightly season with pepper. Refrigerate for at least 4 hours or overnight.

Preheat the grill. Take the steaks from the marinade and place them on the grill. Cook them for 6 to 8 minutes on each side, depending on the thickness. A meat thermometer inserted into the thickest part of the steak should read 140 degrees F for medium-rare and 160 degrees F for well done.

Put the steaks on a plate and cover them with aluminum foil. Allow them to rest for 10 minutes before serving.

Serves 2

Buffalo Kebabs

Kebabs are nothing more than grilled meat and veggies, and you could certainly cook them in a grill basket. But kebabs are so much more festive, and the food cooks evenly. Substitute any veggie or meat you wish, or even add fruit, such as pineapple and peaches.

- 2 tablespoons olive oil
- Juice and zest of 1 lemon
- 2 teaspoons garlic, minced
- Freshly ground black pepper, to taste
- ½ teaspoon thyme
- 1 pound grass-fed buffalo steak, cut in 2-inch cubes
- 1 cup zucchini, sliced
- ½ cup red onion, sliced
- ½ cup grape or cherry tomatoes
- ½ cup red bell pepper, cut in 1-inch cubes

Mix the oil, lemon juice and zest, garlic, black pepper, and thyme in a shallow dish. Place the steak in the dish and refrigerate it overnight.

Drain the marinade and thread the steak on the kebabs with the vegetables. Preheat the grill. Grill the kebabs for 7 to 12 minutes, or until meat is cooked through and the veggies are tender.

Serves 4

Paleo Beef and Broccoli

Restaurant-style beef and broccoli is full of MSG, sodium, and preservatives, but this version is Paleo-approved. Heat the oil until it is almost smoking before you add the beef for a true stir-fry effect.

- 2 tablespoons olive oil
- 1 pound grass-fed flank or round steak, cut in thin strips
- 1 onion, sliced
- 1 pound broccoli florets
- Freshly ground black pepper, to taste
- ½ cup beef stock
- ½ cup low-sodium tamari sauce
- 1 teaspoon garlic, minced
- ½ teaspoon ginger powder
- ½ teaspoon red pepper flakes
- 1 tablespoon quick-cooking tapioca

Heat the olive oil in a large skillet over medium-high heat. Add the steak and cook it quickly, stirring constantly. Transfer the steak to a bowl and add a bit more oil if necessary. Add the onion and broccoli into the pan and cook it quickly, stirring constantly as well. Season with freshly ground black pepper.

Mix the remaining ingredients in a small bowl. Pour the sauce in the pan and cook it until slightly thickened, stirring constantly. Add the beef to the sauce and serve.

Serves 4

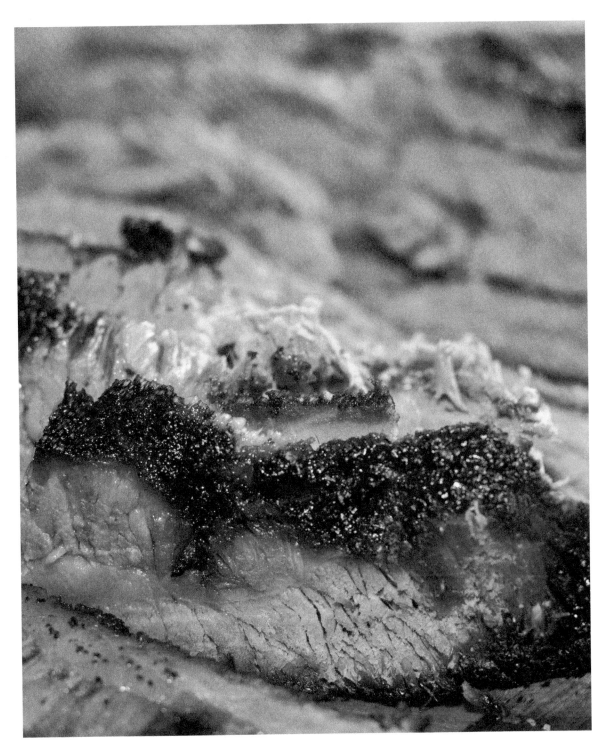

Tangy Beef Brisket (page 118)

Tangy Beef Brisket

Beef brisket comes from the chest of the cow, and is tough and stringy. However, it's reasonably priced and has a lot of flavor. The secret is long, slow cooking. The acid in the tomato paste helps to tenderize this beef brisket, while the molasses gives it some sweetness.

- 1 (6-ounce) can tomato paste
- 2 tablespoons molasses
- 2 tablespoons cider vinegar
- 1 teaspoon dry mustard
- 1 teaspoon garlic, minced
- 2 tablespoons olive oil
- 2 pounds grass-fed beef brisket
- ½ cup onion, chopped
- Freshly ground black pepper, to taste

Mix the tomato paste, molasses, vinegar, mustard, and garlic in a bowl.

Heat the oil in a large skillet over medium heat. Add the beef brisket and brown it on all sides, about 10 minutes. Add the onions and cook until tender.

Transfer the brisket and onions to a slow cooker. Spoon the tomato mixture over the brisket. Season with freshly ground black pepper. Cook on low, 6 to 8 hours, until tender.

Serves 6

Classic Swiss Steak

Swiss steak brings to mind images of June Cleaver in her apron, but it really deserves more attention. This clever dish uses braising to tenderize tough pieces of meat, making them flavorful and delicious. Serve it with braised cabbage or a green salad.

- 2 tablespoons olive oil
- 2 pounds grass-fed beef chuck, cut into 3-inch chunks
- ½ cup onion, chopped
- ½ cup celery, chopped
- 1 tablespoon garlic, minced
- 2 carrots, peeled and sliced
- 1 (14-ounce) can diced tomatoes with the juice
- 1 cup beef broth
- 1 teaspoon paprika
- 1 teaspoon thyme
- 2 tablespoons molasses
- Freshly ground black pepper, to taste

Heat the olive oil in a large skillet. Brown the meat and transfer it to a slow cooker. Sauté the onion, celery, and garlic in the same pan until tender. Transfer to the slow cooker as well.

Add the remaining ingredients to the slow cooker and cook on low until tender, 6 to 8 hours.

Season with freshly ground black pepper. Serve hot.

Serves 4

Buffalo Chili

Rich and meaty, this will be one of your go-to recipes when you want a hot bowl of comfort on a cold night. Even better the next day, you'll be sorry when this is gone. In fact, it's best to plan a day ahead, as the flavors only get better as they meld. Either way, it's still a fantastic and filling meal you'll make time and time again.

- 3 slices uncured, nitrate-free, thick-cut bacon, diced
- 2 pounds grass-fed buffalo, cut into ½-inch chunks
- 1 onion, diced
- 1 green bell pepper, diced
- 2 tablespoons chili powder
- ½ teaspoon cayenne pepper
- ½ teaspoon paprika
- 2 bay leaves
- 1 (15-ounce) can diced tomatoes
- 1-2 cups beef broth
- Freshly ground black pepper, to taste

In a large Dutch oven or stockpot, cook the bacon until crisp. Add the buffalo and brown on all sides. Remove from pot and set aside.

In same pot add onion and bell pepper, cooking until soft. Add seasonings and bay leaves. Add the meat back in the pot.

Pour in the tomatoes and the broth. Season with freshly ground black pepper. Bring to a boil. Simmer for 2 to 3 hours, or until the beef is tender. Simmer longer if you have the time for more flavor.

Serve piping hot.

Serves 6

Chimichurri Strip Steaks

If you're looking for an easy way to add a lot of flavor to steaks, chops, or fish, chimichurri sauce is an excellent choice. It comes together in a flash and gives a flavor profile that is hard to find elsewhere. If you have leftover sauce, you can use it on eggs or fish, or even as a marinade.

- 1 large bunch flat leaf parsley
- 4 cloves garlic, roughly chopped
- Juice of two lemons
- ½ cup olive oil
- ¼ teaspoon red pepper flakes
- Freshly ground black pepper, to taste
- 4 grass-fed New York strip steaks
- Freshly chopped parsley, for garnish

In a food processor, blend the parsley, garlic, lemon juice, and olive oil until smooth. Stir in the red pepper flakes. Season with freshly ground black pepper.

Preheat a gas or charcoal grill to high heat. Grill the steaks until desired doneness, or roughly 6 minutes per side.

When steaks are done, drizzle them with the chimichurri sauce and serve immediately with chopped fresh parsley if desired.

Serves 4

Balsamic Buffalo Tenderloin Steaks

Tenderloin steaks are the most prized cuts of meat available, and buffalo tenderloin is no exception. It's usually served rare to medium rare, but you can cook it to your desired doneness. The tangy balsamic flavor of this tender steak will make you feel like you are in a five-star restaurant, especially if you serve it with grilled or roasted asparagus.

- 1 tablespoon Dijon mustard
- 1 teaspoon ground ginger
- 1 teaspoon garlic powder
- 1 teaspoon onion powder
- 1 teaspoon cumin
- 1 tablespoon balsamic vinegar
- Freshly ground black pepper, to taste
- 4 grass-fed buffalo tenderloin steaks
- 2 tablespoons olive oil
- Freshly chopped parsley, for garnish

Combine all ingredients except olive oil, parsley, and steaks in a small bowl and brush over the steaks. Season with freshly ground black pepper to taste. Heat a large skillet over medium-high heat and add the olive oil. Add the steaks and sear until browned on both sides, about 5 to 6 minutes per side for medium-rare steaks.

Allow the steaks to rest for 10 minutes before serving. Garnish with parsley and serve.

Serves 4

Bison, Bacon, Lettuce, and Tomato

If you love a classic BLT, then you'll love this easy twist that uses a buffalo burger instead of bread. In the summer, these work great on the grill, but you can cook them on a pan for a quick lunch or dinner.

- 8 slices uncured, nitrate-free, thick cut bacon
- 1 pound grass-fed ground bison
- 1 teaspoon garlic powder
- 1 teaspoon onion powder
- Freshly ground black pepper, to taste
- 1 large tomato, sliced
- Butter lettuce

Cook the bacon in a skillet until crispy. Set aside.

Preheat grill if using. In a large bowl, mix the bison with the seasonings, being careful not to overwork. Season with freshly ground black pepper. Shape into 4 patties.

Grill the burgers for about 5 minutes per side, until charred and cooked through.

To serve, top the burgers with the tomato slices, bacon, and lettuce, and eat with a knife and fork.

Serves 4

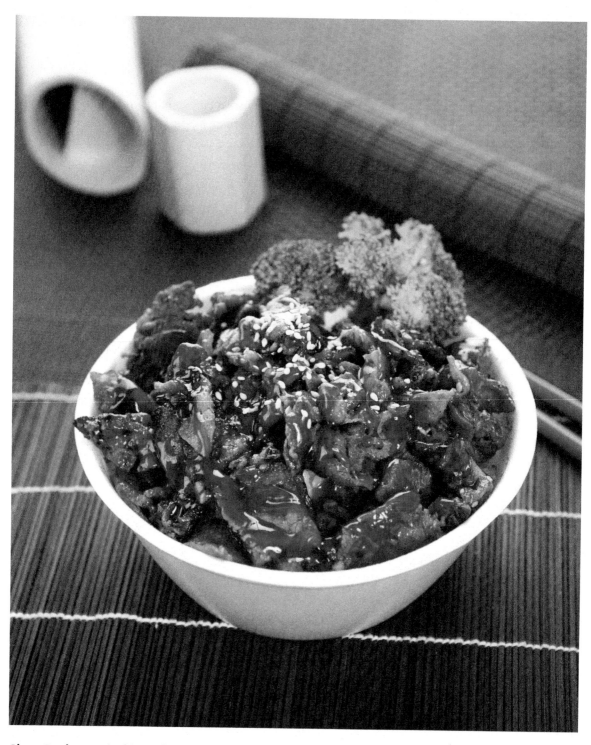

Slow Cooker Teriyaki Beef

Slow Cooker Teriyaki Beef

The sugars in the honey become caramelized as this beef cooks, resulting in a sweet, tender, and highly flavorful meat. Serve it with stir-fried vegetables for a quick meal after work.

- 1 pound grass-fed flank steak or top sirloin, sliced thinly
- ¼ cup coconut aminos
- 1 tablespoon honey
- ½ teaspoon dried ginger
- 1 tablespoon tapioca
- Freshly ground black pepper, to taste
- 1 green onion, chopped

Place the steak in the slow cooker and turn on low.

Mix the aminos, honey, ginger, and tapioca in a bowl. Season with freshly ground black pepper. Pour this mixture over the steak and cover. Cook for 5 to 7 hours, or until very tender. Top with the green onions and serve.

Serves 4

Hungarian Beef Stew

Warm up a cold night with this hearty beef stew. It has more color and flavor than a traditional beef stew, thanks to the addition of bell peppers and tomato paste.

- 2 tablespoons olive or coconut oil
- 1 pound grass-fed beef stew meat
- 1 onion, chopped
- 1 red or yellow bell pepper, seeded and chopped
- 2 cans diced tomatoes
- 1 cup water
- 1 small can tomato paste
- ½ teaspoon paprika
- ½ teaspoon thyme
- ¼ teaspoon crushed red pepper
- Freshly ground black pepper, to taste

Melt the oil in a large saucepan over medium heat. Add the stew meat and cook until browned, turning to brown all sides of the meat. Add the onion and bell pepper and continue cooking an additional 5 to 8 minutes, or until the vegetables are tender.

Stir in the remaining ingredients and bring to a boil. Lower the heat to medium-low, cover and simmer for 45 minutes, or until tender. Season with freshly ground black pepper. Serve hot.

Serves 4

Zesty Meatloaf

Traditional meatloaf recipes call for breadcrumbs or crackers to bind the meat. This delicious alternative uses potato starch instead.

- 2 strips uncured, nitrate-free bacon, diced
- ½ cup onion, diced
- ½ cup red bell pepper, diced
- 1 pound grass-fed ground beef
- 1 large egg

- 2 tablespoons potato starch
- Freshly ground black pepper, to taste
- ½ cup ketchup
- 1 teaspoon dry mustard
- 1 tablespoon maple syrup

Preheat oven to 375 degrees F. Heat a skillet over medium heat. Add the bacon and cook for 4 to 5 minutes, or until brown and crisp. Transfer to a plate with a slotted spoon. Cook the diced onion and bell pepper in the bacon drippings until tender.

Combine the ground beef, egg, and potato starch in a medium bowl. Add the bacon, onions, and bell pepper, and stir gently to mix. Season with freshly ground black pepper. Pour the mixture into a loaf pan.

In another bowl, stir the ketchup, mustard, and maple syrup together. Pour this mixture over the meatloaf. Bake for 40 minutes, or until cooked through and brown on top.

Serves 4

Tangy Marinated London Broil

By marinating these steaks in a flavorful balsamic dressing, you're getting something rich and zesty that's also easy to prepare. The steaks can marinate up to 24 hours before cooking, so be sure to take advantage of that and plan in advance for best results.

- ¼ cup olive oil
- 2 tablespoons balsamic vinegar
- ½ small red onion, minced
- 2 cloves garlic, minced
- 1 tablespoon Dijon or spicy brown mustard
- Freshly ground black pepper, to taste
- 1 pound grass-fed London broil

Combine all ingredients except for the steaks in a gallon-size freezer bag. Put the London broil in the bag and chill for up to 24 hours, making sure the steak is nicely coated.

When you're ready to cook, preheat gas or charcoal grill to high heat. Put the steaks on the grill and cook for about 5 minutes for the first side. Flip and cook another 6 minutes or so until steaks are done.

Allow to rest for 5 to 10 minutes before slicing and serving.

Serves 4

Broiled Lime Rib Steaks

With a variety of spices and seasonings, the smell of these mouthwatering steaks cooking will fill your kitchen and your taste buds with delight. If you have any leftover marinade, you can boil it down for a delicious sauce to use on chicken, pork or any cut of steak.

- 2 cloves garlic, minced
- 1 shallot, minced
- Juice of 1 lime
- 1 tablespoon smoked paprika
- 1 tablespoon cumin
- ½ cup olive oil
- Freshly ground black pepper, to taste
- 2 grass-fed rib steaks

Put the garlic, shallot, lime juice, and seasonings in a food processor and puree until smooth. Slowly drizzle in the oil until you have a smooth and somewhat creamy looking marinade. Season with freshly ground black pepper.

Pour the marinade over the steaks, either in a gallon freezer bag or casserole dish, and chill for 2 to 4 hours.

When ready to cook, preheat broiler on high heat. Put a rack about 6 inches from the broiler.

Put the steaks on a broiler pan and pour any remaining sauce over top of the steaks. Broil for 8 minutes, flip the steaks and broil for 8 more minutes.

Allow to rest for about 5 minutes before serving.

Serves 2

Grilled Stuffed Banana Peppers

These spicy peppers may look like an appetizer, but they make a delicious main course when served with some veggies or a salad. Easy to prepare, these make a unique and interesting meal when you are looking for something besides the same old chicken breasts or pork chops.

- 1 pound grass-fed ground beef
- 2 cloves garlic, minced
- ½ medium onion, minced
- 8 large banana peppers, tops removed, seeds reserved
- Freshly ground black pepper, to taste

In a medium skillet over medium heat, cook the ground beef until browned and cooked through. Add the garlic, onion, and hot pepper seeds. Remove from heat and allow the beef to cool. Lightly season with freshly ground black pepper.

Preheat a grill to high heat. While waiting for the grill to heat up, carefully stuff the peppers with the ground beef mixture. Don't overstuff.

Carefully lay the peppers on the grill (or alternately place foil on grill grates to avoid meat spilling out of the peppers), and grill for about 10 minutes, turning twice throughout the cooking process.

Serve immediately.

Serves 4

Curried Steak Skewers

Warmly spiced, these steak kebabs have a flavor all their own. You can serve these with a vegetable or salad of your choice for a complete meal, or just lay them on a platter and have them as an appetizer for a barbecue. Either way, both you and anyone else you serve them to will think they are delicious.

- 4 grass-fed steaks, cut into cubes
- Juice of 1 lemon
- 1 tablespoon olive oil
- 1 tablespoon cinnamon
- 1 teaspoon curry powder
- 1 teaspoon ground ginger
- Freshly ground black pepper, to taste

If using wooden skewers, soak them for an hour before using.

Put the cubed steak along with the rest of the ingredients in a gallon freezer bag and shake to coat. Marinate and chill for at least 1 hour, and up to 12.

When ready to cook, preheat a grill to high heat. Thread the steaks onto skewers and grill for about 15 minutes, turning every few minutes until steaks are done. Serve with choice of side.

Serves 4

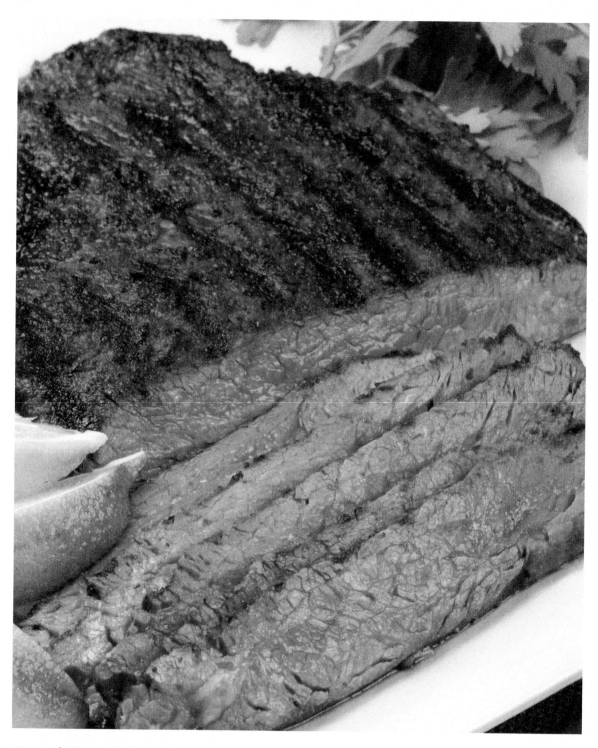

Roasted Citrus Flank Steak

Roasted Citrus Flank Steak

Flank steak can be mouthwateringly delicious when done well, and this recipe does just that. The citrus marinade tenderizes an otherwise tough cut of meat, turning it into a succulent cut that pairs beautifully with simple grilled or steamed vegetables.

- Juice of 1 orange
- Juice of 3 limes
- 2 cloves garlic, minced
- 1 tablespoon Dijon mustard
- 1 tablespoon raspberry vinegar
- 2 pounds grass-fed flank steak
- Freshly ground black pepper, to taste

Combine the orange juice, lime juice, garlic, mustard, and vinegar in a gallon-size freezer bag. Add the flank steak and toss to coat evenly. Chill in the refrigerator for 1 hour.

Preheat oven to 400 degrees F. Lay the steak on a baking sheet or casserole dish and roast for 10 to 12 minutes. Remove from oven and allow to rest for 10 minutes before slicing and serving.

Serves 4

Flank Steak Salad with Sweet Pepper Salsa

This salad is a great example of how flavorsome a meal can be while staying true to Paleo principles. A variety of fresh vegetables and the lean protein from the tasty flank steak are a great combination, and although it is known as a tough cut, flank steak can be tender when sliced thinly across the grain.

- 8 ounces grass-fed flank steak
- 2 sweet bell peppers, seeded and diced
- 2 tablespoons apple cider vinegar
- ½ small red onion, chopped
- 1 small bunch of cilantro, chopped
- 1 red onion, thinly sliced
- 1 large tomato, cut into 8 wedges
- 6 cups mixed baby greens
- Freshly ground black pepper, to taste

Preheat a gas or charcoal grill over high heat. Trim excess fat from steak. Grill steak for approximately 4 to 5 minutes on each side. (It is recommended that flank steak never be cooked past medium-rare or it will become tough.)

Let steak rest for about 5 minutes. While it's resting, prepare the salsa by combining bell peppers, vinegar, chopped onion, and cilantro in a small bowl.

In a large bowl, add salad greens, tomato, and onions.

Then mix in half the salsa mixture and toss well. Season with freshly ground black pepper.

Add the steak to the completed mixtures. Serve warm.

Serves 2

Stuffed Filet Mignon

There is not a more succulent meal on earth than a melt-in-your-mouth, tender fillet mignon topped with sautéed onions and mushrooms. This meal delivers, only with the surprise twist of the savory mushroom and onions stuffed inside the tender cuts of steak.

- 1 tablespoon olive or coconut oil
- 1 small onion, thinly sliced
- 1 cup button mushrooms, thinly sliced
- 2 cloves garlic, minced
- 1 tablespoon balsamic vinegar
- Freshly ground black pepper, to taste
- 2 thick-cut grass-fed tenderloin fillets

Heat a skillet over medium heat. Add the oil, followed by the onions and mushrooms. Sauté for 10 minutes until onions are clear and mushrooms are softened and lightly browned. Add the garlic and cook for another 2 minutes. Add the balsamic vinegar and set aside. Season with freshly ground black pepper.

Preheat a grill over medium-high heat. Cut a small pocket in the side of each fillet, being careful to leave about a half inch between the outside of the steak and the pocket.

Stuff the steaks with the onion and mushroom mixture. Grill for about 5 to 6 minutes per side, or until desired doneness.

Let rest for 5 minutes and serve.

Serves 2

Poultry

Crunchy Pecan Chicken

Forget breaded chicken breasts! Pecan chicken is infinitely better, with a sweet and crunchy crust that the whole family will love. This recipe is easy enough for a weeknight, but elegant enough for a special dinner. Serve it with roasted asparagus or Brussels sprouts for a healthy meal that will become a regular in your menu rotation.

- 4 tablespoons olive or coconut oil
- 2 tablespoons honey
- 1 cup almond meal
- ½ cup pecans, finely chopped
- ½ teaspoon thyme
- ½ teaspoon rosemary
- 4 boneless, skinless chicken breasts
- Freshly ground black pepper, to taste

Preheat oven to 350 degrees F.

Combine oil and honey in a shallow bowl and set aside. Combine almond meal, pecans, thyme, and rosemary in another shallow bowl.

Season the chicken with freshly ground black pepper.

Dip the chicken in the oil and honey mixture, followed by the pecan mixture, coating each piece well.

Place the chicken on a baking dish and bake for 30 to 45 minutes, or until golden brown and cooked through.

Serve immediately.

Serves 4

Grilled Zesty Lime Chicken

This chicken is delicious on its own, or makes a great base for a taco salad. The lime marinade tenderizes the chicken and adds flavor, but be sure to allow at least 12 hours for the best effect.

- 4 boneless, skinless chicken breasts
- Juice and zest of 3 limes
- 1 tablespoon honey
- 1 teaspoon fresh ginger, minced
- 1 jalapeño pepper, minced
- ¼ cup onion, finely chopped
- Freshly ground black pepper, to taste

Place the chicken breasts in a shallow dish. Mix the remaining ingredients and pour over the chicken breasts. Cover and refrigerate for several hours, or overnight.

Preheat the grill. Drain the chicken breasts and grill them for 10 to 15 minutes, turning halfway through the cooking time, until the juices run clear.

Serves 4

Caveman Chicken Nuggets

Looking for a Paleo meal to entice your youngest cavemen? These tasty chicken nuggets are full of protein, but lack the sodium and preservatives found in commercial chicken nuggets. They're so good, in fact, you may have to fight your kids for them. Make a few extra and freeze them for easy lunch meals.

- 2 large egg whites
- ½ teaspoon garlic powder
- ½ teaspoon thyme
- ½ teaspoon rosemary
- 1 cup almond meal
- ½ cup pecans, finely chopped
- Freshly ground black pepper, to taste
- 1 pound boneless, skinless chicken breast, cut in 1½-inch cubes

Preheat oven to 375 degrees F.

Place the egg whites in a shallow dish. Mix the dry ingredients and spices in another shallow dish.

Lightly season the chicken pieces and dip the cubes in the egg whites and then the breading, coating them well. Place the chicken nuggets on a baking sheet and bake for 20 to 25 minutes. Serve immediately.

Serves 4

Slow-Braised Chicken with Sweet Potatoes and Fennel

If you're serious about the Paleo diet, you'll want to learn the technique of braising, which is simply cooking meat in liquid to tenderize it. In this recipe, sweet potatoes are paired with fennel. Fennel has a harsh, licorice taste when raw, but becomes mellow and sweet through slow cooking.

- 2 tablespoons olive or coconut oil
- 1 whole chicken, cut into 8 pieces
- 1 teaspoon garlic powder
- ¼ cup shallots, minced
- 1 cup sweet potatoes, peeled and cubed
- 1 cup fennel bulb, peeled, cored, and sliced
- 1 cup chicken broth
- ½ teaspoon thyme
- Freshly ground black pepper, to taste

Heat the oil in a large saucepan. Place the chicken in the oil to brown it. Add the garlic and shallots and cook until tender.

Add the sweet potatoes and fennel and cook an additional 5 minutes.

Turn the heat to medium-low and add the chicken broth and the seasonings. Cover the pan with a lid and cook for 40 minutes to 1 hour. Take the lid off and simmer an additional 10 minutes to reduce the liquid.

Serve immediately.

Serves 4

Paleo Chicken Fajitas

A classic Tex-Mex cuisine loved by kids as well as adults, fajitas are easy to make in large batches and are a quick throw-together dinner. In this recipe, the steak can be served over a corn or flour tortilla, but it is just as tempting and Paleo friendly without them.

- 3 pounds chicken breasts, cut in thin strips
- 3 green bell peppers, sliced
- 3 onions, sliced
- 2 teaspoons oregano
- 2 teaspoons chili powder
- 2 teaspoons cumin
- 2 teaspoons coriander
- 6 cloves garlic, roughly chopped
- Juice of 5 lemons
- Freshly ground black pepper, to taste
- 4 tablespoons olive or coconut oil
- Butter lettuce leaves, intact for serving
- Your choice of toppings: diced tomatoes, fermented pickles, sauerkraut, sliced avocados, salsa, and/or guacamole

Add the chicken, bell peppers, onions, spices, garlic, and lemon juice in a bowl and combine. Season with freshly ground black pepper.

When preparing ahead of time, marinate in the refrigerator for about 4 hours.

Heat a large skillet on medium heat and cook with the oil until the chicken is cooked through and the onion and bell peppers are soft.

Put the hot chicken in a large bowl and allow people to customize their own fajitas on top of lettuce leaves with their favorite toppings.

Serves 5

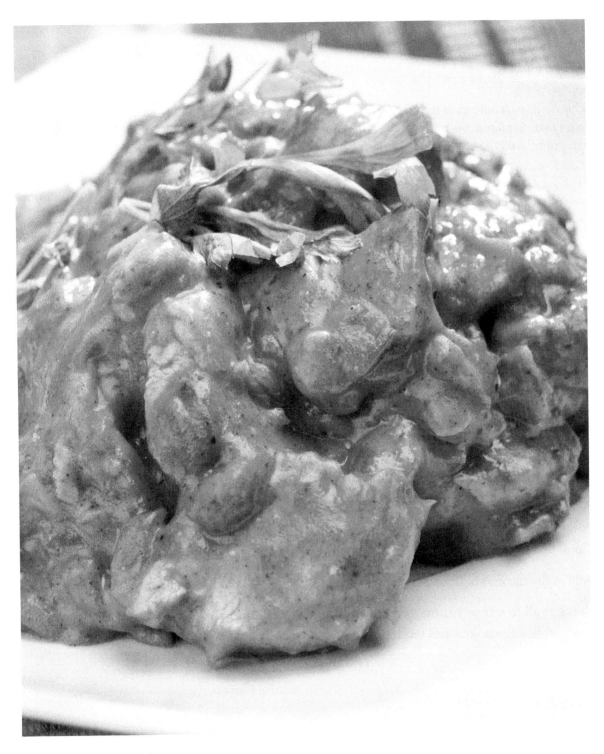

Green Chicken Masala (page 142)

Green Chicken Masala

This recipe may have quite a few ingredients, but it is simple and quick, taking no more than 30 minutes to prepare. Similar to the traditional tikka masala, the combination of Indian spices gives a nice and spicy taste to this dish. You may substitute chicken thighs with pork or beef for equally great results.

- 1 onion, finely chopped
- 3 tablespoons olive or coconut oil
- 2 pounds skinless, boneless chicken thighs, cut into 1-inch pieces
- 1½ teaspoons turmeric
- ¼ cup lemon juice
- ½ cup water or chicken stock
- Small bunch fresh mint leaves
- 2 cups fresh cilantro leaves
- 1 jalapeño pepper, chopped coarsely
- 4 garlic cloves, minced
- ⅛ teaspoon ground cloves
- ½ teaspoon ground cardamom
- ½ teaspoon cinnamon
- 1 cup full-fat coconut milk
- Freshly ground black pepper, to taste

In a large skillet over medium heat, add the onion with the oil. Cook, stirring occasionally for approximately 5 minutes or until the onion starts to soften.

Add chicken thighs and the turmeric to the skillet and continue cooking, stirring occasionally for approximately another 7 minutes.

Place the lemon juice, water or stock, mint, cilantro, jalapeño, and garlic in a blender or food processor and blend until you obtain a smooth puree.

After the chicken has cooked for around 7 minutes, add the cloves, cardamom, and cinnamon. Cook for just about a minute.

Add in the coconut milk, season to taste with freshly ground black pepper and add the herb puree.

Bring it all to a nice simmer and let it continue for approximately 15 minutes, or until the chicken is well cooked and tender.

Serve immediately.

Serves 4

Spicy Chicken with Herb Sauce

This is a simple and scrumptious chicken recipe with chicken rubbed in an unbelievable blend of savory spices and crowned with a sauce of fresh parsley and mint. The key spice here is smoked paprika, made from dried bell peppers that add a touch color and flavor to dishes.

- 2 cups fresh mint leaves
- 1 cup fresh flat-leaf parsley leaves
- 6 cloves garlic, roughly chopped
- 1 green chili, seeded and chopped, optional
- 2 tablespoons Dijon mustard
- 1 teaspoon freshly ground black pepper, to taste

- 1 cup plus additional olive oil
- 2 tablespoons smoked paprika
- 2 teaspoons mustard powder
- 2 teaspoons ground cumin
- 2 teaspoons ground fennel seeds
- 4 boneless chicken breasts

Make the sauce by placing the mint, parsley, garlic, and chili in a food processor and chop roughly. Add mustard, season with pepper and chop again.

Drizzle the 1 cup of olive oil in while the food processor is in a slow mode.

Create the spice rub by combining the paprika, mustard powder, cumin, fennel, and black pepper in a bowl.

Rub the chicken breasts with oil before rubbing them with the spice mixture.

Fry chicken breasts in additional oil for about 5 minutes per side, or until well cooked.

Serve the chicken topped with fresh herb sauce.

Serves 4

Minted Pesto Chicken Stir-Fry

This pleasant blend of mint and pine nuts, stir-fried with tender chicken and mushrooms, adds a very unique idea for your next dinner. Stir-fry is an easy alternative to a heavy meal and can be reheated for a quick lunch.

- 2 cups mint leaves
- ¼ cup toasted pine nuts
- ¼ cup plus 2 tablespoons olive oil, divided
- 1 pound chicken, cut in thin strips
- 1 onion, sliced
- 1 pound mushrooms of any kind, quartered
- Freshly ground black pepper, to taste

Add the mint and pine nuts in a food processor and then slowly add the ¼ cup of oil while pulsing.

Heat the wok and stir-fry the chicken with the 2 tablespoons of oil. Remove chicken from the wok, reheat, and stir-fry the onion for 3 to 4 minutes. Add the mushrooms and stir-fry for another 2 minutes. Season with freshly ground black pepper. Return the chicken to the wok and add in the mint pesto. Cook for another 3 minutes until everything is hot.

Serves 2

Olive, Garlic, and Lemon Chicken

This is an extremely delicious chicken thigh recipe utilizing black olives, garlic, and lemon juice. The merging of those three ingredients, along with the subtle hint of the thyme, makes for an excellent meal that looks sophisticated, but in all reality, is easy to prepare and does not require any special, hard-to-find ingredients. Everything is prepared in a single pan, allowing for quick cleanup afterwards.

- ¼ cup olive or coconut oil
- 8 chicken thighs, with bones and skin
- 3 small onions, thinly sliced
- 3 cloves garlic, minced and smashed almost to a paste
- Freshly ground black pepper, to taste

- 1½ cups chicken stock
- 2 tablespoons fresh thyme, chopped
- ½ cup lemon juice
- ½ pound black olives, cut in half
- 2 lemons, sliced and seeds removed

Preheat oven to 350 degrees F.

Heat oil in a large, hot pan and brown the chicken pieces. Set the chicken aside.

Cook the onions until soft—approximately 3 minutes—making sure to scrape all the delicious chicken bits off the pan while cooking them.

Add the garlic and cook for approximately a minute. Season with pepper.

Add chicken stock, thyme, and lemon juice and return chicken thighs to the pan, skin side up.

Bring to a simmer and then put the pan, covered, in the hot oven for about 20 minutes.

Remove lid and add halved olives and lemon slices. Bake for another 15 to 20 minutes, uncovered.

Serve the chicken with the garlic, olive, and lemon sauce, as well as with some of the lemon slices.

Serves 4

Baked Greek Chicken

Whole chickens are great to use when you are limited on time and need a quick yet healthy meal. The fresh oregano adds a nice authentic Greek taste when mixed with the minced garlic.

- 2 lemons, 1 juiced and zested, 1 peeled
- 3 cloves garlic, minced
- 1 tablespoon fresh oregano, chopped
- Freshly ground black pepper, to taste
- 1 whole broiler chicken, about 5 pounds, cut into 6 pieces
- 1 tablespoon olive oil
- 1 fennel bulb, trimmed, cored, and sliced
- ⅓ cup pitted Kalamata olives, halved

Heat oven to 425 degrees F. In small bowl, mix together 2 teaspoons of lemon zest, 2 tablespoons lemon juice, garlic, oregano, and pepper. Tuck half of this mixture beneath the skin of the chicken.

Cut peel off second lemon and chop fruit into pieces.

Add olive oil to herb mixture in the bowl. Toss with sliced fennel and chopped lemon.

Place in a large baking dish. Top with chicken pieces and bake at 425 degrees F for 40 minutes or until breast meat registers 160 degrees F with an instant-read thermometer. Remove and top with olives.

Serves 4 to 6

Italian Chicken with Dried Oregano

Very simple, and created with ingredients that can be found in your pantry, this recipe has a nice citrus undertone with a strong Italian taste added to the mix. For best results, prepare 8 to 12 hours before cooking to optimize the marinating process.

- 4 pieces of chicken
- 2 tablespoons olive oil
- 2 tablespoons lemon juice
- 1 clove garlic, crushed
- ¼ teaspoon dried oregano
- Freshly ground black pepper, to taste

Mix all of the ingredients in a shallow dish. Turn chicken to coat well. Cover and refrigerate for 8 to 12 hours, remembering to turn it over occasionally.

One hour before serving, heat oven to 450 degrees F. Line a baking sheet with foil, and put chicken on it. Put pan in oven, reduce heat to 325 degrees F. Bake 35 to 45 minutes.

Serves 2

Moroccan Chicken Thighs

A great combination of elements that you would not typically associate with chicken, but that come together nicely to create a wide array of tastes. Easy preparation and simple ingredients make this a great selection for any dinner, but is also just light enough for a Sunday brunch.

- 4 tablespoons olive oil, divided
- 1 small onion, minced
- 1 stalk celery, chopped
- 1 garlic clove, minced
- Freshly ground black pepper, to taste
- 1 large apple, peeled, cored, and diced
- ¼ cup raisins
- ¼ cup walnuts, toasted
- 1 large egg, beaten
- 8 large chicken thighs
- 1 teaspoon allspice

Using a large skillet, heat 2 tablespoons oil. Add onion, celery, and garlic and sauté approximately 3 minutes, or until onion and celery are soft. Season with freshly ground black pepper.

Remove from heat and add apple, raisins, walnuts, and egg. Mix well. Preheat oven to 350 degrees F.

Pull the skin away from the chicken thighs, but do not remove. Stuff apple mixture between the skin and meat. Place chicken in a foil-lined 13 x 9 x 2-inch dish. In a small bowl, add the remaining 2 tablespoons olive oil with allspice and glaze chicken thighs.

Serves 4 to 6

Thai Curry-Braised Chicken

You can control the heat of this dish by the amount of curry paste used. The coconut milk and ginger give it a sweet and spicy taste while creating a full-bodied flavor.

- 4 chicken legs and thighs
- 1 tablespoon olive oil
- Freshly ground black pepper, to taste
- ½ small onion, chopped
- 1 tablespoon fresh ginger, minced
- 2 cloves garlic, minced
- 1 tablespoon Thai red curry paste, to taste
- 1½ cups chicken broth
- 4 bok choy stalks
- 1 cup coconut milk
- Juice of 1 lime
- Fresh chopped cilantro for garnish

Preheat oven to 325 degrees F. Remove the skin from the chicken. Heat the oil in an ovenproof skillet with a lid over low heat. Season the chicken with pepper. Add chicken to the pan and sear on all sides. Take out the chicken and keep warm.

Stir in onions, ginger, and garlic and sauté until onions are soft, approximately 4 minutes. Stir in curry paste along with the broth. Season with freshly ground black pepper.

Place the chicken back in the pan and bring to a simmer. Transfer to oven and cook for 30 minutes.

Cut the bok choy stalks in half and put on a plate with a tiny amount of water, then cover with plastic wrap. Microwave on high for 2 minutes.

Remove pan from oven, remove chicken and reserve. Bring the liquid to a simmer and stir in the coconut milk. Add in lime juice and simmer for 2 minutes. Add the cilantro and return the chicken to the pan.

Place 2 bok choy halves onto each plate. Portion 1 drumstick and thigh on each plate. Spoon sauce over chicken and garnish with more cilantro, if desired.

Serves 4

Spicy Lemon-Turmeric Chicken and Vegetables

Cayenne pepper, ground cumin, and lemon combine in this recipe to create an unforgettable zingy taste that is sure to become a favorite. It does require a bit of cooking time, but you will find that it is worth every moment.

- 1 tablespoon ground cumin
- 1 tablespoon paprika
- 1 tablespoon turmeric
- 1 teaspoon cayenne pepper
- 1 whole lemon
- 3-pound whole chicken
- 1 large onion, diced
- 5 cloves garlic, minced
- ½ cup fresh cilantro, chopped
- 3 large carrots, chopped
- 2 orange bell peppers, seeded and diced
- 1 (14-ounce) can fire-roasted tomatoes, crushed
- 1 tablespoon olive oil
- Freshly ground black pepper, to taste

In a smaller bowl, mix together the cumin, paprika, turmeric, and cayenne pepper. Add the juice from one whole lemon—keep lemon rind—and mix thoroughly.

Using your hands, rub the spice mixture all over the inside and outside of the chicken. Stuff the inside of the chicken with half of the onions, half of the garlic, and half of the cilantro. Set aside.

Place the remaining onions, garlic and cilantro in a 5- or 6-quart slow cooker. Add the carrots, bell pepper, and crushed tomatoes.

Stir in oil. Season with fresh ground pepper. Place chicken on top of the vegetables. Cover and cook on low for approximately 7 hours.

Serve warm.

Serves 4

Slow Cooker Salsa Chicken

When you're pressed for time, the slow cooker can be your best friend. Put a meal in it in the morning, run to work or the store, and by lunchtime, the meal's done. This meal has two ingredients, making it about as simple as can be. Look for organic, natural salsa, which contains minimal amounts of vinegar.

- 2 pounds boneless, skinless chicken breasts
- Freshly ground black pepper, to taste
- 1 (16-ounce) jar salsa

Lightly season the chicken with pepper and place in the slow cooker. Pour the salsa over the chicken.

Cook on low for 4 to 6 hours, or until the chicken is tender and cooked through. Serve with chopped cilantro if you like.

Serves 4

Fruited Stuffed Chicken Thighs

This sweet and savory chicken dish is rich and satisfying, and gets its flavor from apples and raisins, while the walnuts add extra protein and crunch. When served with some steamed veggies or a salad, this becomes a delicious and filling meal.

- 4 tablespoons olive oil, divided
- 1 medium onion, diced
- 1 stalk celery, diced
- 1 garlic clove, minced
- Freshly ground black pepper, to taste
- 2 medium apples, peeled, cored, and chopped
- ¼ cup golden raisins
- ¼ cup chopped walnuts
- 1 large egg, beaten
- 4 large, skin-on chicken thighs
- 1 teaspoon dried tarragon

Preheat oven to 350 degrees F.

Heat 2 tablespoons olive oil in a large skillet over medium heat.

Add the onion, celery, and garlic. Cook for about 4 minutes or until vegetables are tender and translucent but not browned. Remove from heat and season with pepper.

Add apple, raisins, walnuts, and beaten egg. Stir until combined.

Gently pull the chicken thighs apart and stuff the fruit and nut mixture between the skin and meat.

Lay the chicken thighs on a parchment-lined baking pan. Brush the remaining oil over chicken and sprinkle with the dried tarragon.

Bake for 1 hour until chicken is cooked through. Serve immediately.

Serves 4

Garlic Chicken with Mushrooms and Red Peppers

With a spicy and creamy sauce thanks to the coconut milk, you'll be surprised at how flavorful this chicken dish is. Feel free to add whatever veggies you have on hand for variation, or to suit your own personal tastes.

- 4 boneless, skinless chicken breasts, cubed
- 2 tablespoons olive oil, divided
- ½ teaspoon chili powder
- Freshly ground black pepper, to taste
- 1 clove garlic, minced
- 1 medium onion, diced
- 1 cup sliced button mushrooms
- 2 medium red bell peppers, sliced
- ½ cup canned coconut milk

Put the chicken in a gallon-size freezer bag with 1 tablespoon olive oil and chili powder. Refrigerate for one hour.

Heat a large skillet over medium heat and add the remaining oil. Add the chicken and cook until browned on all sides. Add the onion, mushrooms, and red bell peppers and cook until soft. Season with freshly ground black pepper.

Add the coconut milk and simmer until chicken is cooked through and sauce is slightly thickened, about 10 minutes.

Serves 4

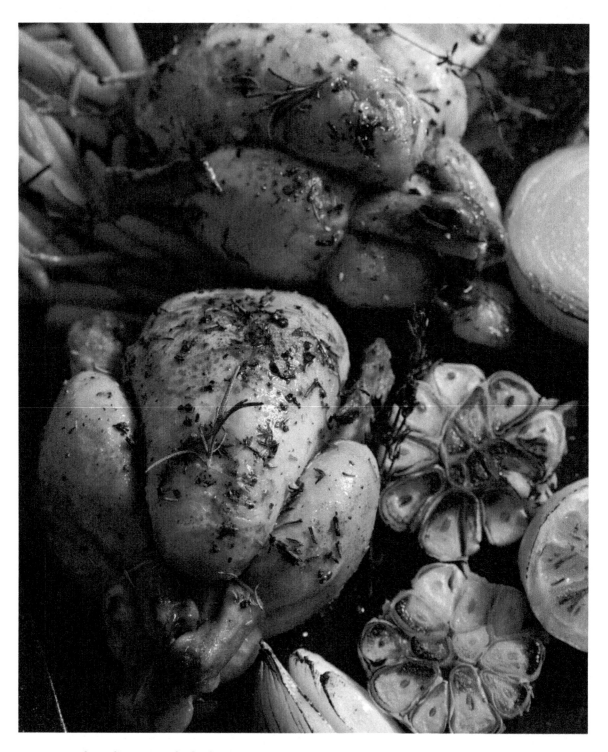

Lemon and Garlic Roasted Chicken

Lemon and Garlic Roasted Chicken

There is nothing much more elegant or delicious than a properly roasted chicken. While it can be intimidating the first time you do it, the truth is that it's much simpler than you think, and can be done for a regular weeknight meal. This lemon and garlic version is mouthwateringly succulent. Once you try it, it will surely be in your regular dinner rotation.

- 1 whole chicken
- 1 lemon
- 2 cloves garlic, minced
- 1 tablespoon fresh rosemary, chopped
- Freshly ground black pepper, to taste
- 2 tablespoons olive oil

Preheat oven to 350 degrees F.

Clean the chicken by removing the giblets and neck and rinsing the entire chicken. Dry thoroughly with paper towels. Put the chicken in a roasting pan, breast side up.

Zest the lemon. Combine the garlic, rosemary, lemon zest, black pepper, and olive oil in a small bowl and brush the mixture over the entire chicken, including inside the bird.

Slice the lemon and stuff the slices inside the cavity of the chicken.

Roast for 25 minutes per pound until the breast temperature reads 170 degrees F on an instant-read thermometer.

Allow chicken to rest for 10 minutes before carving and serving.

Serves 4

Herbed Chicken Kebabs

Chicken is one of the most versatile proteins you can eat, as it takes on many flavors extremely well, including this simple herb mixture. Whether you are grilling these for a quick dinner or making them for a backyard get-together, you'll love the tender and juicy herbed chicken breast pieces.

- 2 pounds chicken tenders
- ¼ cup herbs de Provence
- ¼ cup olive oil
- Zest of one lemon
- Freshly ground black pepper, to taste

Cut the chicken tenders into large chunks, making sure to remove the tendons as you go.

Combine the herbs, oil, and lemon zest in a medium bowl and add the chicken pieces to it. Season with freshly ground black pepper. Allow to chill and marinate for 2 hours before grilling.

When you're ready to cook the chicken, preheat a gas or charcoal grill over medium-high heat.

Thread the chicken onto skewers and grill for 12 to 14 minutes, turning every couple minutes until chicken is browned and cooked through. Serve immediately.

Serves 4

Baked Chicken Thighs

When choosing pieces of chicken, many people automatically choose breast meat because it's lower in fat, but it's also lower in flavor. Luckily, on the Paleo diet you can enjoy any cut of meat you like, including delicious chicken thighs like these. Remarkably simple, these chicken thighs come together beautifully and pair well with just about any vegetable you can think of.

- 4 bone-in, skin-on chicken thighs
- 1 shallot, minced
- 2 cloves garlic, minced
- Freshly ground black pepper, to taste

Preheat oven to 425 degrees F.

Carefully separate the skin from the chicken thighs and stuff the shallots and garlic under the skin. Lightly season the chicken with freshly ground black pepper. Lay on a sheet pan and bake for about 45 minutes, until skin is crispy and the juices run clear. Serve immediately.

Serves 2

Super Garlicky Chicken

This is a variation of the popular "chicken with 40 cloves of garlic" dish that makes many people ask, "How many garlic cloves was that again?" While this version doesn't call for any specific number of cloves, you should use 3 or 4 entire bulbs, not only to get the aromatic garlic flavor, but also so that you can enjoy the delicious steamed cloves themselves, as they are a treat in their own right.

- 1 roasting chicken
- 3 tablespoons olive or coconut oil
- 3 to 4 bulbs of garlic, cloves separated with the skin left on
- Freshly ground black pepper, to taste
- 2 stems fresh rosemary, needles pulled off
- 2 tablespoons fresh thyme, chopped
- 1 shallot, minced

Preheat oven to 350 degrees F.

Cut the chicken into 8 pieces. Heat a large skillet over medium heat and add the oil. Sear the chicken on all sides until browned and crisp, cooking in batches if necessary. Remove the chicken and add the garlic cloves. Cook until browned and remove from heat.

Put half of the garlic cloves in the bottom of a large Dutch oven or soup pot. Season with pepper. Add the chicken and the rest of the garlic on top, followed by the herbs and shallots.

Cover and bake for 90 minutes. Serve immediately.

Serves 4

Maui Chicken

Canned pineapple adds sweetness to this delicious but easy chicken dish. Serve it with roasted vegetables for a quick weeknight meal. Alternatively, place the ingredients in a slow cooker and cook on low for 5 to 6 hours.

- 2 tablespoons olive or coconut oil
- 4 boneless, skinless chicken breasts, cut into 1-inch pieces
- Freshly ground black pepper, to taste
- ½ teaspoon thyme
- 1 (8-ounce) can unsweetened pineapple chunks
- 2 tablespoons quick-cooking tapioca
- 1 teaspoon Worcestershire sauce
- 2 teaspoons Dijon mustard
- 1 green onion, chopped
- ½ cup slivered almonds

Heat the oil in a large skillet. Add the chicken breasts and sauté for 10 minutes, or until tender. Sprinkle the pepper and thyme over the chicken breasts.

Drain the pineapple and set aside, reserving the pineapple juice. In a small bowl, mix together the pineapple juice, tapioca, Worcestershire sauce, and mustard. Pour this mixture into the chicken and simmer over medium-low heat for 10 minutes, or until it thickens slightly.

Top with the pineapple chunks, onions, and almonds to serve.

Serves 4

Maple Walnut Chicken

Maple and walnut create perfect harmony in this classic comfort dish. While maple syrup isn't technically a Paleo staple, there's just enough in this dish to give it the perfect amount of flavor, but not enough that it will ruin your diet. Serve with a large salad for a complete meal.

- 1 tablespoon olive oil
- 1 tablespoon fresh thyme
- ¼ teaspoon freshly ground black pepper
- 4 boneless, skinless chicken breasts
- ½ cup walnuts, chopped
- ⅓ cup apple cider vinegar
- 3 tablespoons pure maple syrup
- ½ cup water

Combine the olive oil with the thyme and pepper.

Rub mixture all over the chicken and let stand for 30 minutes.

While waiting, toast walnuts in a non-stick skillet over medium-low heat for 4 to 6 minutes.

Remove walnuts, add chicken, and turn up the heat to medium. Cook until chicken is done, about 12 minutes, turning once.

Remove chicken to a serving plate.

Whisk the vinegar into the chicken drippings, then add the maple syrup and water.

Simmer for a few minutes until it thickens, add walnuts, then pour over chicken and serve.

Serves 2

Blackened Chicken

No, the chicken isn't burnt—the spices here just darken on the grill. The result is heavenly, with a barbecued chicken that has a deep, intense flavor. If you don't have a grill or want to cook inside, a cast iron skillet will give you a nice charred crust that will match or beat the flavor of the grill.

- 5 pounds chicken thighs and drumsticks
- 1 tablespoon ground rosemary
- 2 tablespoons paprika
- 1 tablespoon garlic powder
- 1 tablespoon onion powder
- 1 teaspoon cayenne pepper
- Freshly ground black pepper, to taste

Mix all of the spices together and rub the chicken all over with it. Heat up a gas or charcoal grill. Place chicken in low heat spots and cook until done.

Spices will blacken but retain their rich flavors. Serve immediately.

Serves 2

Pesto Chicken Pasta with Pistachios

Pistachios are substituted for more traditional pine nuts in this pesto dish, resulting in a sweeter, nuttier flavor. Served with spaghetti squash and sun-dried tomatoes, there is a variety of flavors here, all of which match perfectly.

- 1 medium spaghetti squash, halved, seeds and excess threads removed
- 1 cup pistachios, unsalted and shelled
- 1 cup basil leaves
- 2 garlic
- ½ cup plus additional olive oil
- Juice of 1 lemon
- Freshly ground black pepper, to taste
- 1 pound boneless chicken, sliced or cubed
- Handful of sun-dried tomatoes, sliced, to garnish

Preheat oven to 400 degrees F.

Place spaghetti squash on a baking sheet, cut side down and bake in oven for 25 minutes or until soft.

Pulse pistachios in a food processor 3 or 4 times.

Add basil and garlic and pulse again until you have a chunky mixture.

Turn food processor on and drizzle in olive oil until you get the consistency you want for your pesto.

Add the lemon juice, black pepper and a couple tablespoons of olive oil to a sauté pan and heat over medium-high heat.

Add the chicken.

When the chicken is almost cooked through, add the pesto to the pan. Coat the chicken in the pesto and turn heat down to low. Use a fork to pull the threads out of the cooked spaghetti squash. Add the squash to the pan and mix thoroughly.

Heat through and transfer to a serving bowl. Top with sun-dried tomatoes and enjoy.

Serves 4

Tandoori Style Chicken

This Indian dish has a very appetizing aroma to it and tastes even better. Lots of flavor from spices, paprika and curry infuse the tomatoes and chicken. This is a highly flavorful dish that will satisfy your craving for a meal that's not bland or boring.

- 4 boneless chicken breasts
- 2 cloves garlic, crushed
- 2 bay leaves, finely crushed
- 1 tablespoon tomato puree
- 1 cup canned coconut milk
- 2 tablespoons olive or coconut oil
- 2 tablespoons paprika
- 1 teaspoon curry powder
- Juice of ½ lemon
- Freshly ground black pepper, to taste

Preheat oven to 350 degrees F.

Score the chicken with a knife and place in a baking dish.

Mix together the garlic, bay leaves, tomato puree, and coconut milk. Whisk in the oil and pour mixture over chicken.

Bake for 45 minutes.

Pour off sauce into a serving bowl.

Sprinkle paprika and curry powder over chicken and return to oven for 10 minutes. Season with freshly ground black pepper.

Serve chicken hot with sauce on the side.

Serves 2

Buffalo Chicken Skewers

These will remind you of the wings at your favorite bar, but they are much healthier for you. If you can make your own hot sauce, they'll be even more out of this world, but in a pinch the bottled variety works well. These make great appetizers for a backyard barbecue.

- 5 pounds boneless chicken breasts
- ¼ cup olive oil
- Zest of one lemon
- 1 cup hot sauce
- Freshly ground black pepper, to taste

Soak wooden skewers in water.

Cut chicken into large 1-inch cubes.

Combine olive oil, lemon zest, and hot sauce in a bowl. Season with pepper.

Toss marinade with the chicken and chill for 3 to 4 hours. Preheat a charcoal grill or gas grill to medium-high.

Skewer the chicken and grill until done, about 12 minutes, turning every few minutes to avoid burning.

Serves 5 to 6

Gingery Orange Chicken

Ginger and orange are perfect for chicken. The taste of this dish has a complexity to it as well as just a hint of sweetness.

- 3 pounds chicken legs and/or thighs
- Freshly ground black pepper, to taste
- 2 tablespoons olive oil
- 2 cloves garlic, finely chopped
- 1 cup orange juice
- 2 navel oranges, peeled and sectioned
- 2 tablespoons fresh ginger, minced
- 1 teaspoon dried basil
- Juice of 1 lime

Season chicken with pepper.

Add olive oil to a large sauté pan over medium heat. Add chicken and brown thoroughly (10 to 15 minutes).

Add garlic and lightly brown for 1 minute. Pour in orange juice. Add orange sections, ginger, basil, and lime juice.

Cover and simmer for about 30 minutes or until the chicken is cooked through.

Serves 4

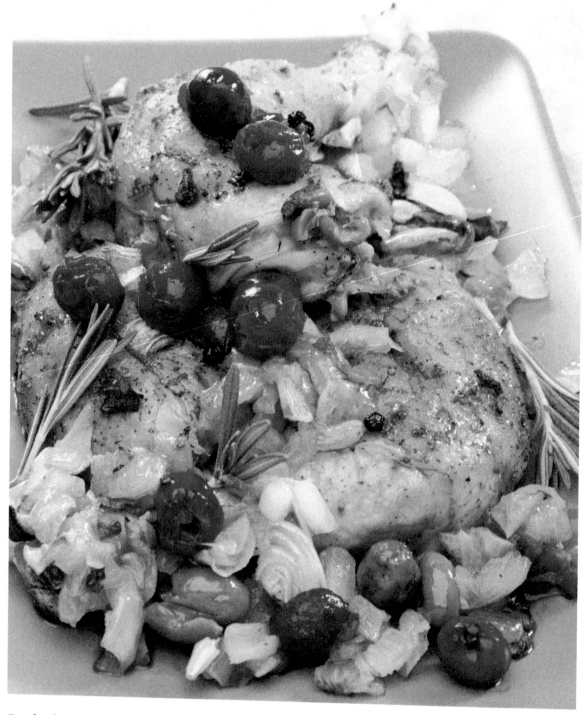

Fresh Cherry and Herbs Chicken

Fresh Cherry and Herbs Chicken

A variety of herbs give this chicken dish an amazing flavor. Lots of fresh cherries and almonds push it over the top. This chicken dish is savory, sweet, and crunchy all at the same time.

- 2 tablespoons olive oil, divided
- 2 shallots, thinly sliced
- 2 cups cherries, pitted and halved
- ⅛ cup red wine vinegar
- ¼ cup balsamic vinegar
- 2 teaspoons cinnamon
- 2 tablespoons dried tarragon
- 1 teaspoon ground ginger
- ½ teaspoon dried oregano
- ½ teaspoon dried thyme
- Freshly ground black pepper, to taste
- 1 pound chicken thighs
- 1 cup sliced almonds

Add 1 tablespoon olive oil to a large sauté pan over medium heat. Stirring occasionally, cook the shallots until translucent (3 to 4 minutes).

Add the cherries, vinegars, cinnamon, tarragon, ginger, oregano, thyme, and pepper. Turn heat down low and simmer for 10 minutes.

Meanwhile, heat another pan over medium-high heat with the remaining tablespoon of oil.

Add the chicken and cook until done (about 12 minutes), turning once.

Heat up a small sauté pan and add the almonds.

Toast the almonds, constantly shaking the pan, until they are lightly toasted and you can smell them.

Divide the chicken among dinner plates.

Pour the sauce over the chicken and garnish with the sliced almonds.

Serves 4 to 5

Duck Breasts with Peach Salsa

If you've never had duck breast, you may be surprised that it doesn't "taste like chicken." In fact, it's in a class all its own. Rich and flavorful, duck has more fat than chicken, but you don't have to worry about that on the Paleo diet.

- 4 duck breasts
- 2 tablespoons olive oil
- Freshly ground black pepper, to taste
- ½ teaspoon thyme
- ½ teaspoon rosemary
- 2 ripe peaches, peeled and chopped
- ½ cup red onion, minced
- ½ cup red bell pepper, chopped
- 1 jalapeño pepper, chopped
- ½ cup fresh mint, chopped
- ½ teaspoon garlic, minced

Preheat the grill. Place the duck breasts on the grill and cook them for 8 to 15 minutes, turning halfway through the cooking time. Meanwhile, mix the olive oil, black pepper, thyme, and rosemary together and brush on the duck breasts as they cook.

Mix the remaining ingredients in a mixing bowl to make the peach salsa. Serve the duck breast with the salsa on the side.

Serves 4

Rosemary Roasted Turkey Breast

While many herbs will complement poultry such as turkey, rosemary adds an extra special distinct flair that is hard to get elsewhere. Serve this moist and tender turkey breast alongside sweet potatoes and a green vegetable for a healthy meal that is reminiscent of the holidays.

- 2 tablespoons olive oil
- 6 pounds organic turkey breast
- 2 tablespoons fresh rosemary, chopped
- Freshly ground black pepper, to taste

Preheat oven to 325 degrees F.

Brush the olive oil over the turkey breast and sprinkle with the fresh rosemary and pepper. Put the turkey breast in a roasting pan and place in the oven.

Roast for about 25 minutes per pound or until an instant-read thermometer reads 170 degrees F.

Allow turkey to rest for 10 minutes prior to slicing and serving.

Serves 8

Turkey Breast with Apples and Sausage

Boneless turkey breasts are a boon to the busy cook. Just roast them in the oven or slow cooker for delicious results.

- 1 tablespoon olive or coconut oil
- 4 nitrate-free breakfast sausage links, cut in 1-inch pieces
- 2 baking apples, peeled and quartered
- 1 boneless turkey breast
- ½ cup apple juice
- ½ teaspoon thyme
- Freshly ground black pepper, to taste

Preheat oven to 350 degrees F. Heat the oil in a roasting pan. Add the sausage and cook 2 to 5 minutes, or until the sausage is browned. Add the apples and cook 3 to 5 minutes, or until the apples are tender. Place the turkey breast on top of the sausages and apples. Add the remaining ingredients.

Roast for 1 to 2 hours, or until the turkey's juices run clear. Alternatively, place the sausage and apples in a slow cooker and add the turkey, apple juice, and seasonings. Cook on low for 6 to 8 hours.

Serves 4 to 6

Turkey Meatloaf

A nice variation on traditional meatloaf, this ground turkey alternative is tasty and easy to put together. While it takes a full hour to bake, the prep is minimal, so a little bit of planning will allow you to have a delicious home dish any night of the week, not just Sunday!

- 2 pounds ground turkey breast
- 1 large egg, beaten
- 1 teaspoon garlic powder
- ½ medium onion, chopped
- 1 small green bell pepper, diced
- 3 stalks celery, diced
- Freshly ground black pepper, to taste

Preheat oven to 375 degrees F.

Using your hands, combine all of the ingredients in a large bowl, being careful not to over mix.

Lightly grease a loaf pan with olive or coconut oil and press the meat mixture into the pan.

Bake for 1 hour, remove, and allow to rest for 15 minutes. Slice, serve, and enjoy!

Serves 6

Lamb

Lamb Chops with Mint Sauce

Lamb chops have a distinctive taste and a rich, succulent texture unlike anything else. Consider lamb chops as a substitute for ham in the spring—or anytime of the year.

- 4 lamb chops
- ½ cup chicken broth
- 1 teaspoon fresh ginger, minced
- 1 teaspoon garlic, minced
- ⅛ cup cider vinegar
- ½ cup mint leaves, finely chopped
- Freshly ground black pepper, to taste

Preheat the grill. Grill the lamb chops for 8 to 10 minutes, turning them halfway through the cooking time.

Mix the remaining ingredients in a saucepan and cook until heated through. Serve on the side with the lamb chops.

Serves 4

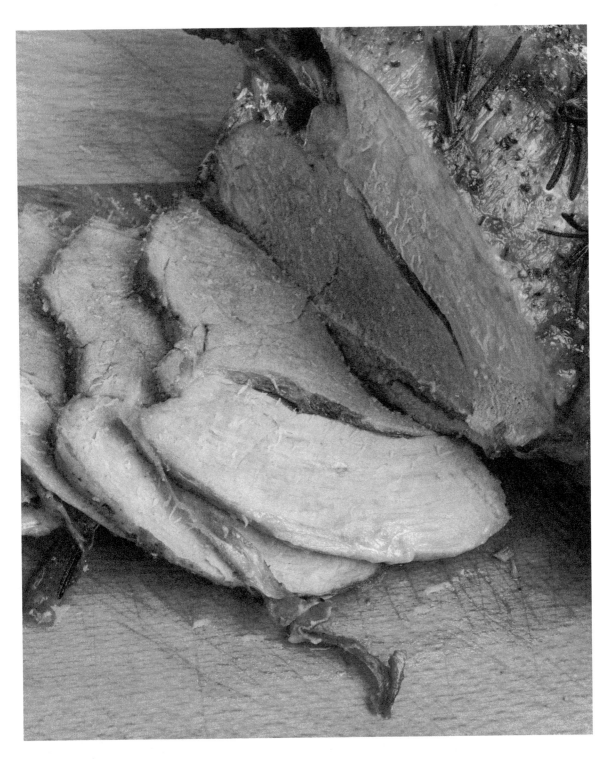

Leg of Lamb (page 174)

Leg of Lamb

Lamb is something typically served in the spring around the Easter holiday, but it's actually a meal that doesn't have to wait for a holiday celebration to be enjoyed. With only a few ingredients, you can enjoy this delicious dish anytime you want and still stick to your diet!

- 3 to 4 pounds leg of lamb
- 1 garlic bulb, separated and peeled
- 2 tablespoons fresh thyme, chopped
- Freshly ground black pepper, to taste

Preheat oven to 325 degrees F. After peeling garlic cloves, push them into lamb leg all over. Rub the thyme all over the lamb leg and lightly season with pepper.

Roast for about 25 minutes per pound for medium-rare, or longer if desired. Allow to rest for 10 to 15 minutes before serving.

Serves 6 to 8

Mediterranean Meatballs with Mint Pesto

This is a variation on traditional Italian meatballs, and one that you'll love. The zucchini "pasta" absorbs the flavors of the mint pesto nicely and complements the hearty flavor of the meatballs.

Mint Pesto:
- 1 large bunch fresh mint leaves
- ¼ cup walnuts
- ½ cup olive oil
- Juice and zest of 1 lemon
- Freshly ground black pepper, to taste

Meatballs:
- 1 pound ground lamb
- 1 teaspoon garlic powder
- 1 teaspoon dried oregano
- 1 large egg, beaten

Pasta:
- 2 large zucchini
- 1 tablespoon olive oil
- 2 cloves garlic, minced

To make the pesto, put all ingredients in a food processor and process until smooth. Set aside.

Preheat oven to 350 degrees F. To make the meatballs, combine the lamb with the spices and egg in a large bowl, being careful not to over mix. Season with pepper. Form mixture into meatballs about the size of a golf ball and place on a parchment-lined baking sheet. Bake for about 25 minutes.

While meatballs are baking, make the zucchini noodles by slicing the zucchini lengthwise into ultra thin noodles. Heat a skillet over medium heat and sauté the garlic for 1 minute in the oil. Add the zucchini and cook until soft and the same texture and consistency of noodles.

To serve, top the zucchini with the meatballs and pesto and garnish with fresh mint if desired.

Serves 4

Mediterranean Lamb Burgers

If you're looking for a delicious alternative to traditional beef burgers, you should try ground lamb. It goes nicely with the mint in these burgers. Serve with a Greek salad for a full meal.

- 1 pound ground lamb
- 2 cloves garlic, minced
- 1 shallot, minced
- 1 small bunch fresh mint, chopped
- Lettuce, sliced tomato, sliced cucumber for serving
- Freshly ground black pepper, to taste

Preheat a gas or charcoal grill to medium-high heat. Using your hands, mix the ground lamb with the garlic, shallot, and mint. Season with freshly ground black pepper. Form into 4 equal sized patties.

Grill the burgers for about 4 to 5 minutes per side until done.

Serve with fresh veggie toppings and a Greek salad for a perfect summer meal.

Serves 4

Lemon and Thyme-Rubbed Lamb Chops

Lemon and thyme complement the richness of lamb very well, which is why you often see these three ingredients together. These chops are simple and form a dish that will liven up any summertime barbecue.

- 2 tablespoons chopped fresh thyme
- Juice and zest of 1 lemon
- ½ cup olive oil
- 6 lamb chops
- Freshly ground black pepper, to taste

Put all ingredients in a gallon-size freezer bag and toss to coat the lamb chops evenly with the marinade. Chill and marinate for at least 1 hour, but up to 24.

When ready to cook, preheat grill over medium-high heat. Grill on both sides until chops are cooked to desired temperatures.

Allow to rest for 10 to 15 minutes before serving.

Serves 2

Grilled Lamb Chops

If you're looking for something different to throw on the grill on a hot summer's night, why not try lamb chops? They're a great alternative to the usual chicken breasts or steaks. This version, with a simple garlic and lemon marinade, is easy to make and super delicious.

- ¼ cup olive oil
- 2 tablespoons lemon juice
- 3 cloves garlic, minced
- 1 small shallot, minced
- 1 teaspoon dried oregano
- Freshly ground black pepper, to taste
- 6 lamb chops

In a small bowl, combine the olive oil, lemon juice, garlic, shallot, and oregano. Season with freshly ground black pepper. Stir to combine well.

Put the lamb chops and the marinade in a gallon-size freezer bag and shake. Chill for at least 1 hour, and up to 24.

When ready to cook, preheat grill to high heat. Grill the chops for about 5 minutes per side. Allow to rest for 10 minutes and serve.

Serves 2

Pork

Pork Medallions with Dried Cherries

Pork medallions are simply pork tenderloins that have been cut into 3-inch slices. They cook quickly and make a great addition to the Paleo diet. For this recipe, you'll brown the medallions and then make a quick reduction, or sauce. A delicious dinner in less than 25 minutes.

- 2 tablespoons olive oil
- 2 pounds pork loin, cut into medallions
- Freshly ground black pepper, to taste
- 1 teaspoon garlic, minced
- ½ cup chicken stock
- ½ cup organic white wine
- 1 teaspoon thyme
- ½ cup dried cherries

Heat the olive oil in a large skillet over medium-high heat. When it is quite hot, but not smoking, add the pork medallions. Cook them for 6 to 10 minutes, turning halfway through the cooking time, until they are well browned. Sprinkle the medallions with pepper and add the minced garlic.

Pour the chicken stock and white wine in the pan. Scrape the bits of meat off the bottom of the pan. Add the thyme. Turn the heat to medium-low and simmer for 10 to 20 minutes, until the meat is cooked through and the sauce is reduced slightly and thickened.

Add the dried cherries and cook an additional 2 minutes.

Serves 4

Sausages with Parsnip Mash and Mushrooms

Bangers and mash are a characteristic English dish, but you don't have to overindulge in potatoes to take pleasure in some appetizing mash. Sweet potatoes, or parsnips, are a perfect substitution. This meal is higher in carbs than most Paleo recipes, but from a natural source and in a reasonable quantity, so it won't be a problem. This meal is particularly good as an after-workout meal, or when you need some fast energy to get you through the day.

- 2 pounds parsnip, coarsely chopped
- 5 tablespoons olive or coconut oil, divided
- ½ cup coconut milk
- Pinch of nutmeg
- Freshly ground black pepper, to taste

- 12 large, good quality beef or pork sausages
- 1 pound button mushrooms
- 2 garlic cloves, minced
- 2 tablespoons

Boil the parsnips for approximately 15 minutes or until soft.

Drain the water and add 2 tablespoons of oil, coconut milk, pinch of nutmeg, and pepper. Mash well with a potato masher. Reserve in the covered pot so they stay warm.

Heat a large skillet over medium heat and cook the sausages with 1 tablespoon of the oil for about 15 minutes, flipping occasionally.

Set sausages aside and add the mushrooms to the already hot skillet with the garlic and the rest of the oil. Cook until well browned, approximately 5 minutes, then add the chopped oregano.

Serve the mashed parsnips smothered with the sausages, mushrooms, and all the drippings.

Serves 6

Pork Chops with Caramelized Apples and Onions

Apples have always been a good match for pork, particularly around the time of year when they are on hand, local and fresh. When plain pork chops served with a side of vegetables don't do it for you anymore, this recipe will remind you of the scrumptiousness of savory pork and sweet apples.

- 4 bone-in pork chops
- Freshly ground black pepper, to taste
- 3 tablespoons olive or coconut oil, divided
- 2 large onions, thinly sliced
- 4 apples, sliced and cored

Season the pork chops with pepper to taste. Heat a large pan over a medium-high heat, add 2 tablespoons of the oil and fry the chops, about 5 minutes on each side or until well cooked and browned.

Set the pork chops aside and reduce the heat to medium-low, then add the remaining tablespoon of oil, as well as the onion and apple slices.

Cook for about 4 minutes, or until the onions have caramelized and the apple slices are softened.

Serve the chops with the topping of apple and onions.

Serves 4

Nectarine and Onion Pork Chops

Apples are frequently coupled with pork, but other fruits can do a noble job, too, as the nectarines do in this recipe. Try out a variation of different fruits with the recipe, such as grapes or berries.

- 3 nectarines, pitted and chopped
- 1 large onion, cut into quarters
- 2 tablespoons olive or coconut oil
- Freshly ground black pepper, to taste

- 6 bone-in pork chops
- Juice of 1 lemon
- 1 tablespoon Dijon mustard
- 1 small bunch fresh mint, chopped

Combine the nectarine and onion in a bowl with the oil and season the mixture to taste with freshly ground black pepper.

Heat a large skillet over medium heat, put in the nectarine and onion mixture and cook, stirring frequently or until the nectarine pieces have softened, approximately 8 minutes.

Set aside to cool. Wipe the skillet clean to cook the pork chops.

Rub additional oil on the pork chops on both sides and season them to taste with pepper. Reheat skillet to a medium heat. Add the chops to the hot skillet and cook for about 3 minutes per side or until well cooked.

When the pork chops are cooking, cut the cooked nectarine and onion quarters into ¼-inch thick slices. Place the slices back into the bowl with their juices.

Mix the lemon juice, mustard, and chopped mint into the nectarine and onion mixture.

Serve the cooked pork chops topped with the nectarine mixture.

Serves 6

Spicy Pulled Pork

Pulled pork is a beloved dinner across America and is created from a slow-cooked pork shoulder or butt roast, with the tender cooked meat pulled apart in shreds. Both pork shoulder or butt roasts are cheap cuts of meat and are a great way to enjoy appetizing meat when on a budget— especially when feeding large groups of people.

- 3 tablespoons smoked paprika
- 1 tablespoon garlic powder
- 1 tablespoon dry mustard
- 1 pork shoulder or butt roast, about 5 to 6 pounds
- 1½ cups apple cider vinegar
- ½ cup ketchup
- 1 cup Dijon mustard
- 2 garlic cloves, minced
- 1 teaspoon cayenne pepper
- ½ teaspoon freshly ground black pepper

Prepare dry rub by combining the paprika, garlic powder, and dry mustard in a bowl.

Rub the pork roast with the spice rub and put in the refrigerator for the flavors to penetrate the meat for a minimum of 1 hour, or overnight for best results. If marinating only for 1 or 2 hours, leave the roast at room temperature.

Preheat oven to 300 degrees F.

Put the marinated pork shoulder or butt in the oven on a baking pan for approximately 6 hours, until the meat is falling off the fork.

Prepare the sauce by mixing the apple cider vinegar, ketchup, Dijon mustard, garlic, cayenne pepper, and black pepper in a small pot or saucepan.

Smoothly bring to a simmer, stirring occasionally, and simmer for approximately 10 minutes.

When the pork roast is ready, remove from the oven and let cool for 10 minutes.

Pull the meat apart from the roast with two forks.

Combine the spicy sauce with the pulled pork and serve with favorite side or salad.

Serves 8 to 10

Cilantro Pork Stir-Fry

Cilantro and pork go extremely well together. The lime juice added near the end also supports the cilantro and adds a very unique taste.

- 4 garlic cloves, finely chopped
- 1 tablespoon ginger, finely chopped
- ¼ cup olive oil
- 1 bunch of cilantro, chopped
- 1 pound tender pork, thinly sliced

- 2 medium onions, thinly sliced
- Freshly ground black pepper, to taste
- 1 red bell pepper, thinly sliced
- Juice of 1 lime

Combine the garlic, ginger, olive oil, and half the cilantro in a bowl. Add the pork and place in the refrigerator to marinate for an hour or two. Heat wok and stir-fry the pork.

Remove the pork, add more oil and stir-fry the onions for approximately 3 minutes. Season with freshly ground black pepper.

Add bell pepper and stir-fry for approximately 3 more minutes or until soft. Place the pork back in the wok with the lime juice and the other half of the cilantro leaves and allow to cook for another minute while mixing to blend the flavors.

Serve warm.

Serves 2

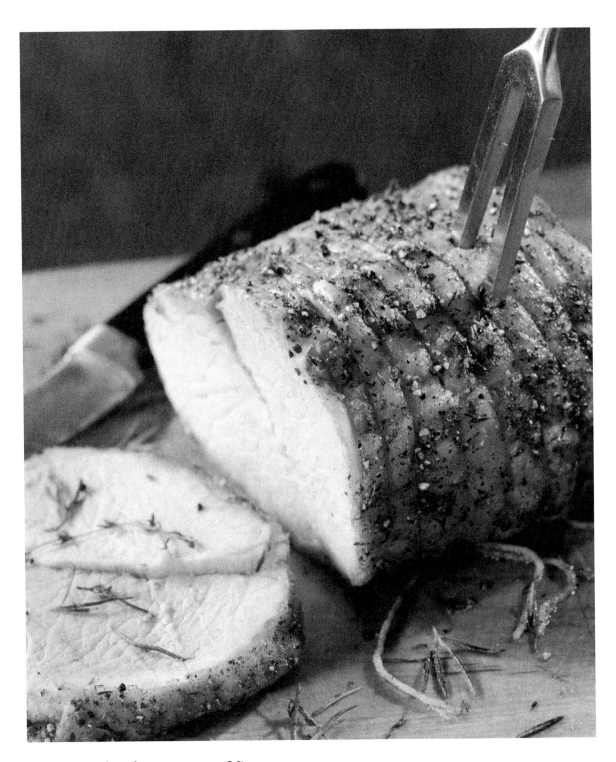

Slow Roasted Pork Roast (page 186)

Slow Roasted Pork Roast

One of the best things about the Paleo diet is that it includes a lot of your favorite comfort foods. (Okay, not all of them, but who needs mac 'n' cheese when you can eat this pork roast?) Serve this with a green salad drizzled with olive oil for a complete and satisfying meal you'll make again and again.

- 2 tablespoons olive oil
- 4-pound pork roast
- 1 small onion, sliced
- 2 garlic cloves, smashed
- 2 sweet potatoes, peeled and diced
- 1 cup tomatoes, diced
- 1 bay leaf
- 2 cups chicken or beef stock
- Freshly ground black pepper, to taste

Preheat oven to 325 degrees F. In a large Dutch oven, add the oil and pork roast. Sear until deeply browned on all sides. Remove and set aside.

Add onions and garlic to the pot and cook until softened. Add sweet potatoes, tomatoes, bay leaf, and stock. Bring to a boil and reduce heat to a simmer. Season with freshly ground black pepper.

Simmer for 2 hours and then turn oven down to 250 degrees F and continue cooking until roast is tender, about 2 to 3 more hours. Serve immediately.

Serves 4 to 6

Maple-Glazed Pork Roast with Sweet Potatoes

Natural maple syrup still contains a lot of sugar, but it's permissible as an occasional treat on the Paleo diet. In this recipe, it creates a delicious glaze for the pork and sweet potatoes, enhanced by orange juice and ginger.

- 2 tablespoons olive or coconut oil
- 1 boneless pork loin roast
- 2 sweet potatoes, peeled and cubed
- ½ cup pure maple syrup
- Zest and juice of 1 orange
- ½ teaspoon ginger
- Freshly ground black pepper, to taste

Heat the oil in a large skillet. Brown the pork roast evenly, 7 to 10 minutes. Transfer the roast to a slow cooker. Add the sweet potato cubes.

Mix the maple syrup, orange juice and zest, and ginger in a bowl. Season with freshly ground black pepper. Pour this mixture over the roast. Set the slow cooker on low and cook for 6 to 8 hours.

Serve the pork with the sweet potatoes on the side.

Serves 4

Savory Sausage

Commercial sausage is full of nitrates, sodium, and preservatives—all no-no's on the Paleo diet. Old-time sausage recipes called for fresh herbs and garlic instead, making a healthy and flavorful alternative. This recipe makes a large batch, enough to freeze for later use. You'll find a million uses for it—from dinner casseroles to savory fruit and meat dishes.

- 3 pounds ground pork
- ½ cup onion, finely minced
- ½ cup Italian parsley, finely minced
- 2 teaspoons garlic, minced
- 2 teaspoons ground ginger
- 2 teaspoons red pepper flakes
- 1 teaspoon ground cloves
- Freshly ground black pepper, to taste

Combine all the ingredients in a large mixing bowl. Use your hands to mix the sausage until well combined. Form the sausage into 3-inch rounds.

Cook the sausage in a skillet over medium heat for 15 to 17 minutes, or until cooked through and browned. Turn halfway through cooking time.

Makes 18 rounds

Sunday Pork Roast

When buying pork roast, opt for a boneless roast with firm, pink flesh and uniform marbling. Serve this tasty pork roast with steamed vegetables and a salad for a complete meal.

- 2 tablespoons olive or coconut oil
- 3-pound pork roast
- ½ teaspoon thyme
- ½ cup apple juice
- Freshly ground black pepper, to taste

Heat the oil in a medium skillet. Add the pork roast and brown the meat on each side to form a savory crust.

Transfer the roast to a slow cooker and add the thyme and apple juice and cook on low for 6 to 8 hours, or until very tender. Season with freshly ground black pepper.

Serve hot.

Serves 4

Slow Cooker Pork Tenderloin and Apples

Pork tenderloin is a delicious protein choice for the Paleo diet. Succulent and sweet, it pairs well with a variety of ingredients. When buying pork tenderloin, look for pork that is light pink with a firm texture. Avoid those that have liquid pooling in the tray or seem spongy. Serve this dish with roasted sweet potatoes and Brussels sprouts.

- 2 tablespoons olive or coconut oil
- 2 pounds pork tenderloin
- Freshly ground black pepper, to taste
- ½ cup chicken stock
- 3 tart apples, peeled and quartered
- 2 tablespoons honey
- 1 teaspoon cinnamon

Add the oil to a large skillet over medium heat. Add the pork tenderloin and brown on all sides.

Transfer the pork tenderloin to a slow cooker. Season with black pepper. Pour the chicken stock over the roast and cook on low for 6 to 8 hours.

Add the apples to the slow cooker. Mix the remaining ingredients in a small bowl and pour over the apples. Cook an additional hour.

Serves 4

Fish and Seafood

Baked White Fish and Mediterranean Salad

You'll find a lot of fish on the Paleo diet—it's good for you, and with a mild white fish there are lots of ways you can cook it. Any mild white fish, such as cod or tilapia, works well here, but feel free to use what you have.

- 2 (6 to 8 ounce) white fish fillets of your choice
- Juice from 1 lemon
- 1 cucumber, diced
- ½ cup black olives
- 1 tomato, seeded and diced
- 1 red onion, sliced
- Olive oil and red wine vinegar, to taste
- Freshly ground black pepper, to taste

Preheat oven to 350 degrees F. Lightly spray a baking sheet with cooking spray. Place fish on baking sheet and drizzle with lemon juice. Bake for 10 to 12 minutes until fish flakes easily with a fork.

Combine cucumber, olives, tomato, and onion in a large bowl. Drizzle with olive oil and vinegar, season with pepper. Divide salad between two plates.

To serve, place the baked fillets on top of the salad.

Serves 2

Pan-Fried Trout with Kale

You'll find trout in most good fish markets these days, although if you can catch it yourself, so much the better! Trout is a fairly lean fish. Nitrate-free bacon adds fat and flavor to this dish and pairs nicely with the kale.

- 2 strips of uncured, nitrate-free bacon
- 2 trout fillets
- 2 cups kale, chopped
- Freshly ground black pepper, to taste
- ½ teaspoon dill
- Juice and zest from 1 lemon

Cook the bacon in a large skillet over medium heat. Transfer it to a plate and crumble it.

Sauté the trout in the bacon drippings until golden brown, firm, and opaque, about 7 to 10 minutes.

Transfer the fish to a plate and keep warm. Sauté the kale in the same pan for 4 to 6 minutes, until limp. Season with freshly ground black pepper and dill. Don't overcook, as this will cause it to become tough and bitter.

Place the kale on two plates and serve the fish over it. Sprinkle all with lemon juice and zest.

Serves 2

Grilled Salmon with Grilled Veggies

Salmon is a meaty fish that performs beautifully on the grill. Just make sure to spray the grill first with a non-stick spray and don't try to turn the fish until it's done. Salmon is cooked when it's firm to the touch and opaque. Don't overcook it, though, which will dry it out.

- 4 salmon fillets
- Freshly ground black pepper, to taste
- Juice and zest from 1 lemon
- 1 cup zucchini, cut in rounds
- ½ cup red bell pepper, chopped
- ½ cup red onion, sliced
- ½ cup carrots, sliced

Preheat the grill. Place the salmon fillets on the grill and dust them with pepper, lemon juice, and zest. Cook for 5 to 8 minutes, turning halfway through. Transfer to a plate.

Place the remaining ingredients in a grill basket and spray with cooking spray. Cook 12 to 15 minutes, or until tender. Stir frequently so the onion doesn't burn. Allow to rest for 5 minutes before serving.

Serves 4

Cod with Sautéed Mushrooms

Fresh cod fillets have a slightly firm texture and a mild, sweet flavor that pairs perfectly with sautéed mushrooms. Serve this delicious dish with steamed vegetables for a quick weeknight meal.

- 4 cod fillets
- 2 tablespoons olive or coconut oil
- ½ cup mushrooms, chopped
- 3 tablespoons full-fat coconut milk
- Freshly ground black pepper, to taste
- ¼ teaspoon dill
- 1 tablespoon lemon juice
- 1 tablespoon dried or fresh parsley

Preheat oven to 400 degrees F. Spray a 9 x 13-inch baking pan with non-stick cooking spray. Place the fish in the pan. Bake 8 to 10 minutes, or until firm and white.

Heat the oil in a small skillet. Add the mushrooms and sauté 5 minutes, or until tender. Add the coconut milk and heat to warm. Season with freshly ground black pepper and dill.

To serve, place a fillet on each plate and drizzle the mushrooms and milk over the fish. Top with lemon juice and parsley.

Serves 4

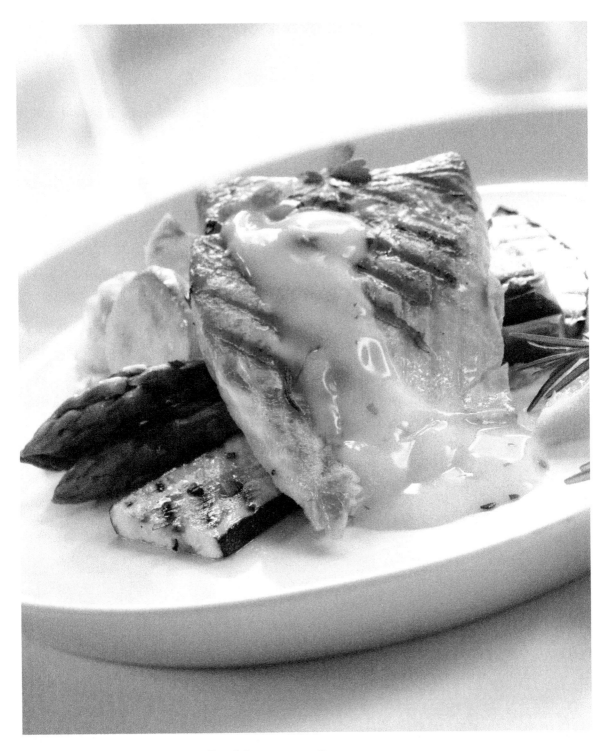

Slow Roasted Salmon with Hollandaise (page 196)

Slow Roasted Salmon with Hollandaise

Hollandaise sauce needs to be served warm, and should be made right before serving it—but it goes together in a snap to give this salmon a creamy finish.

- 14 tablespoons olive or coconut oil
- 4 salmon fillets
- 4 large, cage free, organic egg yolks
- Juice of 1 lemon
- ¼ teaspoon cayenne pepper
- Freshly ground black pepper, to taste

Melt 2 tablespoons of the olive or coconut oil in a large frying pan, reserving the remaining or coconut oil. Place the salmon in the hot frying pan and cook it for 8-12 minutes, turning halfway through the cooking time.

Melt the remaining olive or coconut oil in the microwave. Blend the egg yolks, lemon juice and peppers in a blender. Slowly add the melted olive or coconut oil, a few drops at a time, and continue blending until the mixture emulsifies and becomes thick.

To serve, position the salmon over roasted asparagus or steamed bok choy. Drizzle the dish with the Hollandaise sauce.

Serves 4

Roasted Lemon Pepper Salmon Fillets with Spinach

Salmon is one of the healthiest foods you can eat, as well as being pretty easy and fast to cook. It's high in protein and omega-3 fatty acids. You'll definitely find it on top of most Paleo favorites lists—and for good reason. Not only is it super healthy, it's also delicious. Since you're not loading up on carbs like rice here, it's okay to buy a bigger piece of fish. Along with the wilted spinach, you'll feel full for the rest of the evening.

- 2 (6 to 8 ounce) salmon fillets
- 2 teaspoons lemon pepper seasoning
- 1 tablespoon olive oil
- 1 clove garlic, minced
- 4 cups tightly packed baby spinach

Preheat oven to 400 degrees F. Coat salmon fillets on both sides with the lemon pepper seasoning. Lightly spray a baking sheet with cooking spray and place fillets on top. Roast salmon for about 15 minutes, flipping halfway through, or until fish flakes easily with a fork.

While salmon is cooking, heat oil in a large sauté pan. Add garlic and cook for 30 seconds or so, being careful not to burn. Add spinach and cook until it begins to wilt.

Divide spinach evenly between two plates. Top with the salmon fillets and serve immediately.

Serves 2

Steakhouse Crab Cakes

When you're craving something deep-fried, try these instead. Egg whites give them crunch without a lot of oil, so you can indulge with no guilt. Find flaked crab at your butcher's fish counter.

- 2 tablespoons olive oil
- ½ cup onion, chopped
- ½ cup celery, finely minced
- ½ cup red bell pepper, finely minced
- Freshly ground black pepper, to taste
- 1 teaspoon garlic, minced
- 2 egg whites

- ½ cup almond meal
- ½ teaspoon cayenne pepper
- ½ teaspoon cumin
- ½ teaspoon red pepper flakes
- 1 pound flaked crab
- 1 strip uncured, nitrate-free bacon, cooked and crumbled

Preheat oven to 375 degrees F. Heat the oil in a skillet over medium heat. Add the vegetables and cook until tender. Season with freshly ground black pepper.

Transfer the cooked vegetables to a bowl, and combine them with the remaining ingredients. Shape them into 3-inch rounds and bake for 15 to 20 minutes, or until golden brown.

Serves 4

Offal

Oxtail Stew

If you've never had this hearty and rich dish, you are missing out on a delicious alternative to beef stew. Oxtails are just what they sound like—meat from the tail of a steer—and they can be found in upscale butcher shops, some Asian markets, or sometimes warehouse stores like Costco. It's a very tough cut of meat and needs to be slow-cooked for hours, so make sure you plan ahead before attempting this dish.

- 2 tablespoons olive oil
- 3 pounds oxtails, with separated joints
- 1 medium onion, chopped
- 1 celery stalk, chopped
- 1 large carrot, chopped
- 3 cloves garlic, peeled
- 4 cups chicken or beef stock
- 1 bay leaf
- Pinch of dried thyme
- Freshly ground black pepper, to taste
- 2 carrots, cut into bite-sized pieces
- 2 parsnips, cut into bite-sized pieces
- 2 turnips, cut into bite-sized pieces

Heat a large Dutch oven over medium heat and add the oil. Add the oxtails to the pan and brown on all sides. Remove from pan and set aside.

Add the onions, celery, and chopped carrot to the pan and cook until vegetables are tender, about 10 minutes. Add the oxtails and garlic to the pan, along with the stock. Add the bay leaf and thyme and bring to a boil. Season with freshly ground black pepper.

Reduce heat to low and simmer for about 3 hours, or until the meat is tender.

After the stew has been simmering for 2 hours, preheat oven to 350 degrees F.

Toss the carrots, parsnips, and turnips with a little olive oil and roast on a single layer on a sheet pan for 45 minutes to 1 hour.

When the oxtail meat is tender, skim the fat from the stew. Add in the roasted vegetables and heat for 15 to 20 minutes before serving.

Serves 4 to 6

Calves Liver with Sage

Calves liver is the most tender of all organ meats. It doesn't take long to cook, and has a velvety texture that's hard to find in other cuts of meat. You can use lamb's liver to save money if necessary, but you'll find it's not quite as tender. If you don't love the strong flavor of liver, you can tone it down by soaking it in milk for a few minutes.

- 2 tablespoons olive oil
- 12 fresh sage leaves
- 8 thin slices calves liver
- Freshly ground black pepper, to taste
- Juice of 1 lemon

Heat the oil in a medium skillet over medium-high heat. Add the sage leaves and cook until browned. Remove from pan.

Add the liver slices and cook until browned on all sides. Season with freshly ground black pepper.

Add the sage leaves to the pan, followed by the lemon juice. Cook for 1 minute and serve immediately.

Serves 4

Pan Fried Veal Sweetbreads

Sweetbreads are something that many people are hesitant to taste, but once they do, they can't get enough. Not what the name implies, sweetbreads are actually the thymus gland of the animal, in this case, veal. They are very mild in flavor, but have a rich and velvety texture that makes them a delicacy in foodie circles. If you've never tried them, this simple recipe is a great starter.

- 6 ounces veal sweetbreads
- 1 cup almond or coconut milk
- Juice of 1 lemon
- 2 tablespoons olive or coconut oil
- 1 teaspoon capers
- Freshly ground black pepper, to taste
- Fresh parsley, chopped, for garnish

Soak the sweetbreads in the milk overnight.

Before cooking, discard the milk and rinse the sweetbreads with cold water. Put in a pot, cover with water and add the lemon juice. Bring to a boil and blanche for about 5 minutes. Drain, and dry well.

Heat a large skillet over medium heat and add the oil. Add the sweetbreads and cook until golden brown. Add the capers to the pan, season with pepper, cook for 1 minute, and divide the sweetbreads between two plates.

Serve immediately.

Serves 2

Wild Game

Venison Medallions with Quick Mustard Sauce

If you haven't been around hunters or hunted your own meat, you may have never tried venison, which is deer meat. While it does taste similar to beef in dishes like tacos, it does have a unique flavor that stands out in this dish. If you know a hunter and can get fresh venison, do so; otherwise, meat from a butcher will do.

- 3 tablespoons Dijon mustard, divided
- 1 to 2 pounds venison tenderloin, cut into medallions ½-inch thick
- 1 tablespoon olive or coconut oil, divided
- 1 shallot, minced
- Freshly ground black pepper, to taste
- 1½ cups beef stock

Rub 1 tablespoon of the mustard into the medallions. Heat a large skillet over medium-high heat and add 1 tablespoon of oil. When the pan is very hot, add the venison to the pan, cooking in batches if necessary. Sear for 4 minutes per side and remove from the pan.

Add the remaining oil and shallots to the same pan and reduce the heat, scraping up any browned bits. Season with freshly ground black pepper.

Add the stock and remaining mustard and whisk to create a smooth sauce.

To serve, drizzle the sauce over the venison medallions.

Serves 4

Venison and Pork-Stuffed Peppers

This unique take on traditional stuffed peppers is an excellent choice for a dinner party, as the brightly colored peppers have great visual appeal, and the recipe gives guests who have never tried venison a chance to ease into it. Serve these with a big green salad for a complete and healthy meal that is also super filling.

- 6 bell peppers, whatever colors you prefer
- 4 slices uncured, nitrate-free bacon, chopped
- ½ pound ground pork
- ½ pound ground venison
- 2 stalks celery, diced
- 1 small onion, chopped
- 4 cloves garlic, minced
- 5 green onions, chopped
- 1 small bunch fresh parsley, finely chopped
- 2 large eggs, beaten
- Freshly ground black pepper, to taste

Preheat oven to 350 degrees F.

Cut off the tops of the peppers and remove the seeds and membrane with a pairing knife. Chop the tops and set aside.

Bring a large pot of water to a boil and turn off the heat. Add the peppers and soak for about 5 minutes, no longer.

Heat a large skillet over medium heat and add the bacon. Cook until crispy, then remove from the pan. Add the pork and venison and cook until browned, about 10 minutes. Add the celery, onions, garlic, and reserved chopped peppers. Cook for another 10 minutes and add the green onions and parsley. Transfer mixture to a pan and allow to cool and mix in the eggs. Season with freshly ground black pepper.

Stuff the peppers with the mixture, pressing the meat down into the peppers to assure you have none left over.

Bake in a casserole dish until the tops are browned, about 30 minutes.

Serve immediately.

Serves 6

Roast Loin of Venison

If you enjoy the unique flavor of venison, you'll love this simple roast that doesn't have any competing ingredients. Serve with any vegetable of your choice for a complete meal.

- 4 pounds boneless loin of venison
- Freshly ground black pepper, to taste
- 2 tablespoons olive oil

Preheat oven to 400 degrees F. Lightly season the venison loin with pepper and brush with the oil.

Set the meat in a roasting pan and roast for about 30 minutes for medium-rare, longer if you like it more well done.

Allow venison to rest for 10 minutes before slicing and serving.

Serves 8

Braised Rabbit

Rabbit is a white meat that is very mild, although it does have a flavor all its own. This recipe is an easy way to get the most out of your rabbit and is great for those who have never tried it before. Your butcher will cut your rabbit however you like; in this recipe, it's cut in quarters and braised until tender.

- ¼ cup olive oil
- 3-pound rabbit, cut into quarters
- 1 large onion, sliced
- 3 cloves garlic, minced
- 2 cups chicken stock
- 1 tablespoon fresh thyme, chopped

- 1 bay leaf
- Freshly ground black pepper, to taste
- 1 tablespoon cornstarch mixed with 1 tablespoon cold water
- Juice of 1 lemon

Heat the olive oil in a large skillet over medium heat and add the rabbit pieces. Brown on all sides, remove from pan, and set aside.

Add the onions and garlic and cook until tender, about 3 minutes.

Add the stock, thyme, and bay leaf. Put the rabbit back in the pan and bring to a boil. Season with freshly ground black pepper.

Reduce heat and simmer for 35 to 40 minutes, until tender. Remove rabbit from pan and add cornstarch mixture. Simmer for 5 minutes while whisking. Stir in the lemon juice.

To serve, place the rabbit on plates, and pour the sauce over it.

Serves 4

Fillet of Ostrich with Mixed Mushrooms

Ostrich is very similar to beef in texture, but is leaner, so it's lower in fat. You can get it at a local butcher, but it might be a bit more expensive than beef. While it may not be something you'll eat everyday, it's definitely worth trying, especially in this recipe with mushrooms.

- 1½ tablespoons olive or coconut oil, divided
- ½ pound mixed mushrooms of your choice, sliced
- ½ shallot, minced
- 2 cloves garlic, minced
- Freshly ground black pepper, to taste
- 6 ostrich fillets
- ¼ cup beef stock
- 1 tablespoon tomato paste
- Fresh parsley, chopped, for garnish

Heat a large skillet over medium heat and add ½ tablespoon oil. Add the mushrooms and cook until lightly browned and tender. Add the shallots and garlic and continue cooking about 2 minutes. Season with freshly ground black pepper. Remove from pan.

Add the remaining oil to the pan and add the ostrich fillets. Cook until nicely browned on both sides.

Add the stock and tomato paste, scraping up any browned bits as you cook. Add the mushroom mixture back to the skillet and heat through.

Serve the ostrich topped with the mushrooms and garnished with parsley.

Serves 6

Casseroles

Paleo Lasagna

If you find that you crave pasta on the Paleo diet, you'll be surprised to find that you do have some options. One of them is this delicious lasagna that will satisfy your craving for the comforting casserole. A mandolin will yield the best results as far as the zucchini slices go, but you can slice it with a sharp knife if necessary.

- 1 pound grass-fed ground beef
- 3 cloves garlic, minced
- 1 small onion, chopped
- 1 small green bell pepper, diced
- 6 ounces tomato paste
- 1 (15-ounce) can tomato sauce
- 1 tablespoon fresh parsley, chopped
- 2 tablespoons Italian seasoning
- Freshly ground black pepper, to taste
- 1 large zucchini, thinly sliced lengthwise
- 1 cup mushrooms, sliced

Preheat oven to 350 degrees F. In a large pot over medium heat, brown the beef while continuously stirring.

Add the garlic, onion, and bell pepper and continue cooking for about 5 more minutes.

Stir in the tomato paste and sauce, followed by the herbs. Season with freshly ground black pepper.

Bring to a boil and remove from heat.

In a 9 x 13-inch casserole dish, place a thin layer of the sauce. Layer the zucchini and mushrooms over the sauce and alternate layers until they reach the top or you run out of ingredients.

Cover with foil and bake for 25 to 30 minutes. Remove foil and bake for an additional 5 minutes. Allow to rest for 5 minutes before serving.

Serves 8

Pork and Leek Casserole

This casserole is easy to throw together but makes for a very filling meal. Leeks are a mild member of the onion family, and if you've never had them before, they look like giant green onions. The white parts are the only parts that are edible, so it may seem like a waste, but they are so tender and delicious they are well worth the trouble.

- 2 medium onions, finely chopped
- 3 leeks, cleaned thoroughly and white parts sliced thin
- 1 cup mushrooms, roughly chopped
- 1 tablespoon dried oregano
- 6 pork tenderloin medallions
- 1 cup chicken stock
- 1 (15-ounce) can diced tomatoes
- 1 tablespoon tomato paste
- Freshly ground black pepper, to taste

Preheat oven to 350 degrees F.

Place all of the ingredients into a casserole dish. Cover with the lid or foil.

Bake for 3 to 4 hours or until pork is cooked through.

Place 1 to 2 tenderloins on each plate and spoon vegetables over the top before serving.

Serves 2

Spanish Lamb Casserole

This rich and flavorful casserole dish uses fatty lamb meat with lots of complementing vegetables. Fresh herbs and red wine give this casserole its intense flavor. This is a great alternative to a roast on a spring holiday, or a fitting meal any other time of the year.

- 2 tablespoons olive oil
- 2 pounds lamb meat, legs or chops, whichever you prefer
- Freshly ground black pepper, to taste
- 1 head of garlic
- 2 tomatoes, chopped into 6 to 8 pieces each
- 1 green bell pepper, seeded and chopped
- 1 carrot, chopped into small pieces
- 1 large parsnip, chopped into small pieces
- 1 onion, chopped into small pieces
- 2 sprigs of rosemary
- 1 bay leaf
- 1 cup organic red wine
- 1 cup chicken stock

Cut the lamb meat into 1-inch chunks. Heat the oil in a large sauté pan.

Add the lamb meat, season with pepper and brown on all sides, about 5 minutes.

Add the vegetables to the pan and fry until they begin to brown. Transfer the meat and vegetables to a large casserole dish.

Add the rosemary, garlic cloves, and bay leaf, then pour in the red wine and stock. Season with freshly ground black pepper.

Cover and put in oven for 2 hours. Remove the rosemary sprigs. If the sauce is too thin, return to the oven and let some of the liquid evaporate.

Ladle the meat and vegetables into bowls to serve.

Serves 5 to 6

Chipotle Chicken and Sweet Potato Casserole

This spicy chicken and sweet potato casserole is easy to prepare, full of flavor and sure to be a crowd pleaser. Loaded with veggies, bacon, and hearty chicken, it's also filling enough to be a meal on its own. Bonus: It tastes even better the next day!

- 2 pounds of sweet potatoes
- 2 tablespoons olive oil
- 1 red bell pepper, chopped
- 1 cup green onions, chopped
- 3 cloves of garlic, minced
- 1 teaspoon chili powder
- 1 teaspoon chipotle powder
- ½ teaspoon ground cumin
- 2 chicken breasts, grilled and chopped
- 6 strips of uncured, nitrate-free bacon, cooked and crumbled
- 1 cup cherry tomatoes, chopped
- 3 tablespoon fresh cilantro, chopped
- Freshly ground black pepper, to taste

Cook the sweet potatoes in boiling water until tender.

Let cool slightly, then peel the sweet potatoes and cut into 1-inch chunks. Preheat oven to 375 degrees F.

Add oil to a large pan over medium heat and add the bell pepper and green onion.

Cook for 2 minutes, then add the garlic and sauté for another minute.

In a large bowl, mix together the bell pepper mixture, sweet potatoes, chili powder, chipotle powder, cumin, chicken, bacon, tomatoes, and cilantro. Season with freshly ground black pepper.

Transfer the mixture to a large casserole dish.

Bake for 20 minutes or until everything is heated through. Serve immediately.

Serves 6

Chicken Cauliflower Alfredo Casserole

Casseroles can be hard to come by on the Paleo diet, since most of them are loaded with rice, pasta, or potatoes. This dish is a powerhouse for protein and fat, leaving you feeling extremely full without all those unwanted carbs. Chicken, bacon, eggs, and vegetables give you everything you need for the day, and in a way that is mouthwateringly delicious.

- ½ cup olive or coconut oil
- 1¾ cups full-fat coconut milk
- 1 teaspoon garlic powder
- ½ medium onion, chopped
- 3 large eggs
- Freshly ground black pepper, to taste
- 3 boneless, skinless chicken breasts, cooked and cubed
- 2 cups broccoli crowns, chopped
- 4 cups cauliflower, steamed and chopped
- 6 strips of uncured, nitrate-free bacon, cut into quarters

Preheat oven to 375 degrees F.

Whisk the oil together with the coconut milk, garlic powder, onion, and eggs. Season with freshly ground black pepper.

Add in the chicken, broccoli, and cauliflower and mix thoroughly. Pour into casserole or cake pan. Place bacon in a single layer across the top.

Bake for 1 hour. Then broil for 5 to 6 minutes until bacon is crispy. Allow to rest for 10 minutes before serving.

Serves 4 to 5

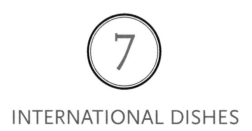

INTERNATIONAL DISHES

Mexican

Caveman Fajitas

The secret to tasty fajitas lies in marinating the meat in a spicy marinade, resulting in a tender, juicy meat that stands well all on its own. Grilling gives the meat and veggies a smoky flavor, although you can prepare them in a skillet, as well.

- 2 tablespoons olive oil
- Zest and juice of 4 limes
- 2 jalapeños, chopped
- 1 (8-ounce) can chipotle chilies
- ½ teaspoon cayenne pepper
- 1 teaspoon garlic, minced
- ½ teaspoon crushed red pepper

- 1 pound grass-fed steak, chicken or fish, cut into 1-inch strips
- 1 onion, cut in small slices
- 1 green bell pepper, cut in rings
- 1 red bell pepper, cut in rings
- Freshly ground black pepper, to taste

Mix the olive oil, lime juice and zest, chilies and seasonings together in a shallow dish. Add the meat and marinate overnight for best flavor. Drain the meat.

Preheat the grill. Place the meat in a grill basket, sprayed with cooking spray, and cook for 5 to 12 minutes, or until tender. Do not overcook. Transfer to a plate. Cook the vegetables for

8 to 12 minutes, until tender, stirring frequently so you don't burn the onions. Season with freshly ground black pepper.

Serve the steak alongside the veggies.

Serves 4

Mexican Chicken Salad

Shredded chicken makes easy work of lunch on the Paleo diet. To make a quick salad, simply add a few vegetables, a protein, and a savory dressing. Switch it up for variety. The basic formula for any salad dressing is simply one part acid to two parts oil. Add seasonings, such as ginger, chilies, garlic, or juice to change the flavor.

- 1 cup chicken breast, cooked and shredded
- ½ cup red onion, chopped
- ½ cup red bell pepper, chopped
- ½ cup avocado, cubed
- ½ cup jicama, julienned
- 4 cups baby salad greens
- ½ cup fresh lime juice, with the zest
- 1 teaspoon garlic, minced
- 1 teaspoon cumin
- ½ teaspoon crushed red pepper flakes
- ½ teaspoon cayenne pepper
- ½ cup cilantro, chopped
- 1 tablespoon honey
- 1 cup grapeseed oil
- Freshly ground black pepper, to taste

Combine the shredded chicken and vegetables in a salad bowl.

Whisk the lime juice, lime zest, garlic, spices, cilantro, and honey together in a bowl. Slowly add the grapeseed oil in a steady stream, whisking vigorously until it emulsifies. Season with freshly ground black pepper. Toss the salad with the dressing and serve immediately.

Serves 4

Asian

Curried Shrimp

This curried shrimp tastes authentically Indian, but requires only a few ingredients and takes less than 25 minutes to prepare. Unless you live in a coastal area, most shrimp in the store has been frozen, including the shrimp labeled "fresh." In most cases, you're better off buying frozen shrimp.

- 2 tablespoons olive oil
- 2 tablespoons green curry powder
- 1 pound broccoli florets
- 3 carrots, peeled and sliced
- 1 (8-ounce) can coconut milk
- 1 pound large shrimp, deveined and shelled
- Freshly ground black pepper, to taste

Heat the oil over medium heat. Stir in the green curry powder and cook for one minute. Add the broccoli, carrots and coconut milk. Cook for 10 to 15 minutes, or until the veggies are tender and the coconut milk becomes thick.

Stir the shrimp in during the last 5 minutes. Overcooking it will cause it to become tough and rubbery. Season with freshly ground black pepper.

Serve immediately.

Serves 4

Garlic Ginger Chicken

This dish has a delicious Asian twist to it with ginger, garlic, fish sauce, and coconut aminos, which is a healthy alternative to traditional soy sauce. You can find them either in a health food store or Asian grocery store.

- 2 tablespoons olive or coconut oil
- 1 tablespoon fresh ginger, minced
- 5 cloves garlic, smashed and minced
- ¼ teaspoon fish sauce
- ¼ cup coconut aminos
- 4 chicken legs
- Freshly ground black pepper, to taste

Preheat oven to 425 degrees F.

Heat the oil in a small saucepan.

Add the ginger, garlic, fish sauce, and coconut aminos and bring to a simmer for 3 minutes.

Put the chicken in a baking dish and pour the sauce over the top. Sprinkle with pepper. Bake for 45 minutes.

Remove and let stand for 10 minutes before serving.

Serves 3 to 4

Green Curry Chicken

This wonderful chicken dish is packed with spices, as well as a large variety of vegetables—onions, eggplant, carrots, cauliflower, zucchini, and mushrooms.

- 2 tablespoons olive oil
- 3 small yellow onions, diced
- 3 cloves garlic, minced
- 1 tablespoon fresh ginger, minced
- 2 pounds chicken thighs
- 1 eggplant, diced
- 3 large carrots, diced
- ½ head cauliflower, cut into 1-inch pieces
- 1 zucchini, diced
- 8 ounces mushrooms, sliced
- 2 cans coconut milk
- 3 tablespoons green curry powder
- Freshly ground black pepper, to taste

In a large pot, heat the oil over medium-high heat. Add the onions, garlic and ginger.

When the onions begin to soften, add the chicken.

Cook for 10 minutes, then add the eggplant and carrots. Cover the pot, and when the eggplant begins to soften add the rest of the vegetables.

After 10 minutes, add the coconut milk and green curry powder. Season with freshly ground black pepper.

Simmer the mixture until the vegetables are soft but not mushy. Serve chicken in a bowl with lots of sauce over the top.

Serves 3 to 4

Chinese Five-Spice Ribs

With the exotic flavor profile from the Chinese five-spice powder and the delicious sesame glaze, these melt-in-your-mouth tender ribs will have you swearing off Chinese takeout for good.

- 6 pounds pork baby back ribs
- 1 tablespoon Chinese five-spice powder
- 1 teaspoon curry powder
- ½ teaspoon coriander
- 3 tablespoons sesame oil
- ½ teaspoon fish sauce
- 2 cloves garlic, minced
- 1 tablespoon fresh ginger, chopped
- Freshly ground black pepper, to taste

Cut the ribs into 6 portions. Bring two large pots of water to boil and boil the ribs for about 30 minutes. Drain and lay on a baking sheet to cool.

Season the ribs with the seasonings and cover with foil. Chill for 1 hour.

Heat a charcoal or gas grill to medium-low heat. Combine the remaining ingredients in a small bowl.

Put the ribs on the grill and grill for about 20 minutes. Baste with the sesame oil glaze and continue cooking for 20 more minutes, basting with any remaining glaze.

Serve immediately.

Serves 6

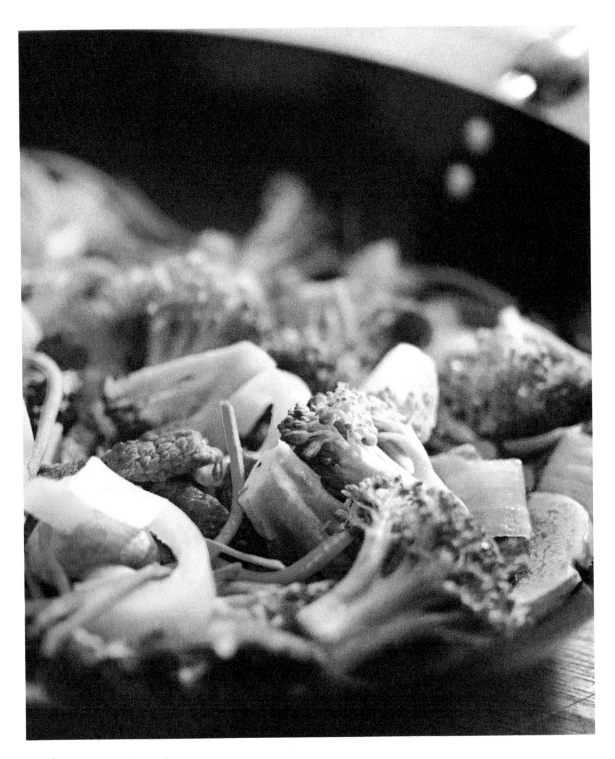

Beef Stir-Fry (page 220)

Beef Stir-Fry

You'll have to eat this stir-fry without rice if you're trying to stick to the diet, but with the flavor from high-quality beef, it's unlikely you'll miss it. As with all cooking, you want to buy the highest quality beef you can find, not only for flavor, but for health reasons as well.

- 1 pound grass-fed beef round, sliced into thin strips
- 2 tablespoons olive oil
- 1 garlic clove, minced
- 1 cup broccoli florets
- 1 cup carrots, sliced
- 1 cup snow pea pods
- ½ head cabbage, finely shredded
- 1 teaspoon apple cider vinegar
- Freshly ground black pepper, to taste
- Sesame seeds for garnish, if desired

Heat a large, non-stick skillet or wok over medium-high heat. Add sliced beef and cook until browned on all sides, almost cooked through. Remove from pan and set aside.

Add oil to pan, add garlic, followed by vegetables and vinegar. Stir-fry until crisp and tender. Season with freshly ground black pepper.

Add beef back to pan and finish cooking. Divide into bowls, top with sesame seeds, if desired, and serve immediately.

Serves 4

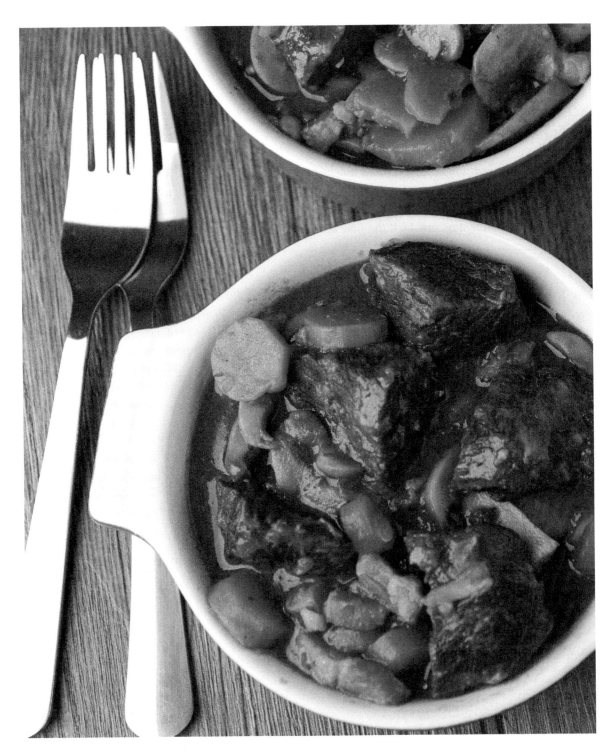

Beef Burgundy (page 222)

French

Beef Burgundy

Beef burgundy is traditionally served with mashed potatoes or noodles, but you won't miss them. This flavorful French stew is teeming with veggies and savory meat. Best of all, it cooks in the slow cooker, making it suitable for even a weeknight meal. Combine the ingredients the night before and refrigerate. In the morning, just turn the slow cooker on and dinner is made.

- 2 slices uncured, nitrate-free bacon
- ½ cup onion, chopped
- 1 teaspoon garlic, minced
- 1 pound grass-fed beef stew meat
- 5 carrots, peeled and diced
- 2 cups beef broth
- 1 cup organic red wine
- 3 tablespoons quick-cooking tapioca
- 3 tablespoons tomato paste
- ½ teaspoon thyme
- Freshly ground black pepper, to taste
- 2 tablespoons olive or coconut oil
- ½ cup mushrooms, chopped

Cook the bacon in a large skillet over medium heat. Crumble and transfer to the slow cooker. Add the onion and garlic to the bacon drippings and cook until tender. Brown the stew meat in the bacon drippings and transfer it to the slow cooker.

Add the carrots, broth, wine, tapioca, tomato paste, thyme, and pepper to the slow cooker. Cook on low for 6 to 8 hours.

Heat the oil in a small skillet and sauté the mushrooms for 5 to 7 minutes, or until tender. Stir the mushrooms into the stew and serve.

Serves 4

Roasted Chicken with Root Vegetables

Roasted chicken is a classic dish that, when prepared correctly, is amazingly delicious. When served with the root vegetables in this recipe, this is a great meal for entertaining. To get perfectly crisp skin on your chicken, allow it to come to room temperature before roasting.

- 1 (4-pound) roasting chicken
- Freshly ground black pepper, to taste
- 6 cloves garlic, smashed
- 2 medium rutabagas, peeled and cut into wedges
- 2 medium turnips, peeled and cut into wedges
- 4 large carrots, peeled and cut into 2-inch pieces
- 1 medium onion, cut into quarters
- ¼ cup plus 4 tablespoons olive oil, divided

Preheat oven to 475 degrees F.

Lightly season the chicken with pepper. Rub the garlic cloves all over the inside and outside of the chicken and stuff them inside the chicken. Truss the chicken legs together with kitchen string.

Put the vegetables in a bowl and toss with the ¼ cup oil. Lay in a roasting pan and put the chicken on the bed of vegetables.

Rub the remaining oil over the outside of the chicken and put the pan in the oven. Roast at 475 degrees F for 25 minutes, reduce heat and roast for 45 more minutes until the thickest part of the thigh registers 160 degrees F on an instant-read thermometer.

Allow the chicken to rest for 20 minutes before carving and serving.

Serves 4

Salmon en Papillote

Don't be fooled by the name. En papillote simply means "in parchment," and it's one of the simplest methods around for cooking fish and other foods. The fish is tucked in a paper pocket and baked in a hot oven. The paper creates a hothouse effect, quickly steaming the food, while keeping it moist. Place one pocket on each plate and snip it open with kitchen shears for a simple, but elegant, presentation.

- 4 salmon fillets
- 1 cup carrots, julienned
- 1 cup asparagus spears, chopped
- 1 cup broccoli florets
- 6 tablespoons olive or coconut oil

- 1 teaspoon dill
- ½ teaspoon minced garlic
- ½ teaspoon thyme
- Juice and zest of 1 lemon
- Freshly ground black pepper, to taste

Preheat oven to 375 degrees F. Place four 12-inch squares of parchment paper on 2 baking sheets. Fold the sheets of parchment paper in half and unfold.

Place a salmon fillet on each sheet of parchment paper, positioning it on one side, so you can fold the paper over. Mound the vegetables on top of the fish.

Mix the remaining ingredients in a small bowl. Place 2 tablespoons of the mixture on top of each pile of vegetables. Season with freshly ground black pepper.

Fold the paper over the top of the vegetables. Starting in one corner, fold the paper down to make a tightly sealed packet. Bake for 12 to 15 minutes.

Serves 4

Italian

Paleo Spaghetti and Meat Sauce

If you haven't tried spaghetti squash, you're in for a treat. The squash has a sweet, mellow flavor and forms spaghetti-like strands when cooked. Serve it with this hearty, slow-cooker meat sauce for a filling lunch or dinner.

- 1 pound grass-fed ground beef
- ½ cup onion, chopped
- ½ cup celery, chopped
- ½ cup carrots, chopped
- 2 teaspoons garlic, minced
- 3 (14-ounce) cans tomato puree
- 1 (8-ounce) can tomato paste
- ½ cup organic red wine
- 1 teaspoon thyme
- 1 teaspoon marjoram
- 1 spaghetti squash
- Freshly ground black pepper, to taste

Brown the ground beef in a large skillet. Add the vegetables and cook them until they are tender. Transfer the ground beef and vegetables to a slow cooker, and add the remaining ingredients except the spaghetti squash.

Preheat oven to 350 degrees F. Cut the squash in half and remove the seeds. Place the squash in a baking pan, cut side down. Fill the pan with 2 inches of hot water. Cover with aluminum foil and bake for 40 minutes, or until tender. Scoop the squash out and place it in a serving dish. Serve with the meat sauce.

Serves 6

Chicken Cacciatore

Here's another slow-cooker recipe for chicken cacciatore, the classic Italian chicken stew. Forgo the breading, and simply brown the chicken, which brings out its flavor admirably. This chicken tastes even better the next day, so make enough for leftovers.

- 2 tablespoons olive oil
- 4 chicken breasts or 1 whole chicken, cut in pieces
- 1 teaspoon garlic, minced
- 1 small onion, cut in rings
- 1 cup green bell pepper, cut in rings
- Freshly ground black pepper, to taste
- 2 (14-ounce) cans diced tomatoes, drained
- 1 (8-ounce) can tomato paste
- 1 teaspoon marjoram

Heat the olive oil in a large skillet. Add the chicken and brown it on all sides, about 10 minutes. Add the garlic, onions, and bell peppers, and cook an additional 5 minutes. Transfer the chicken and vegetables to a slow cooker. Season with freshly ground black pepper.

Add the remaining ingredients and cook on low for 6 to 8 hours. Serve with steamed spaghetti squash for a more traditional Italian meal.

Serves 4

Regional American

Paleo Style Gumbo

Enjoy the authentic flavors of Louisiana cuisine with this rice-less gumbo. Okra and tapioca thicken it slightly, and sautéed onions, peppers, and celery—the holy trinity of cooking—add flavor. Chances are, you'll never miss the rice!

- 2 tablespoons olive oil
- ½ cup onion, chopped
- ½ cup green bell peppers, chopped
- ½ cup celery, chopped
- Freshly ground black pepper, to taste
- 1 cup okra, sliced and chopped
- 4 cups chicken stock
- 1 (14-ounce) can diced tomatoes, drained
- 2 tablespoons molasses
- 2 tablespoons Tabasco sauce
- 2 cups chicken, cooked and shredded
- 1 pound shrimp, cooked
- ½ pound high quality sausage, browned and crumbled

Heat the olive oil in a large stockpot over medium heat. Add the onions, bell peppers, and celery and cook until tender, stirring frequently. Season with freshly ground black pepper.

Add the okra and cook an additional 2 minutes. Stir in the remaining ingredients and simmer for 40 minutes.

Serve immediately.

Serves 6

Southern Style Shrimp

If you've ever been to a crawfish boil, you know how much fun it is. Crawfish, corn on the cob, and red potatoes are boiled in a spicy broth. Once cooked, the contents are thrown on a table covered with newspaper. Crawfish are a bit hard to come by in most parts, but shrimp is just as tasty. You'll love this Paleo-adapted version of a crawfish boil.

- 1 pound shrimp, shells intact
- 2 medium onions, quartered
- 1 cup tomatoes, chopped
- ½ cup fresh cilantro, minced
- 2 teaspoons ground cumin
- ½ teaspoon cayenne pepper
- ½ teaspoon crushed red pepper flakes
- Freshly ground black pepper, to taste

Bring 4 cups of water to a boil in a large pot. Combine all the ingredients in a large bowl, stirring to coat the shrimp well.

Pour the shrimp into a steamer basket and place the steamer basket over the boiling water. If you don't have a steamer, improvise with a metal colander. Place the lid on the pot and steam for 5 minutes. Ladle into 4 bowls and serve.

Serves 4

Pulled Pork with Homemade Barbecue Sauce

Pork roast is delicious cooked in the slow cooker. It becomes moist and savory. Commercial barbecue sauce is laden with high fructose corn syrup, sugar, and vinegar, but this homemade version is much healthier—and just as yummy.

- 2 tablespoons olive oil
- 2-pound boneless pork roast
- 1 teaspoon garlic, minced
- Freshly ground black pepper, to taste
- 1 (28-ounce) can tomato puree
- ½ cup onion, chopped
- ½ cup chicken broth
- ½ cup cider vinegar
- ¼ cup molasses
- 1 teaspoon dry mustard
- ¼ teaspoon ground cinnamon
- ¼ teaspoon ground allspice
- ¼ teaspoon ground cloves
- ¼ teaspoon ground ginger
- ¼ teaspoon ground red pepper flakes

Heat the olive oil in a skillet. Add the pork roast and brown slightly. Browning caramelizes the meat and improves its flavor. Place the pork roast in a slow cooker and add the garlic. Season with freshly ground black pepper. Cook on low for 3 to 4 hours, or until tender. Remove and shred.

Puree the tomatoes and onions in a food processor or blender. Add the pureed tomato and onions and remaining ingredients to the slow cooker, mixing well. Cook an additional 2 hours to meld the flavors.

Serves 4

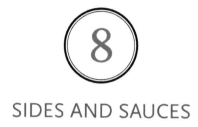

SIDES AND SAUCES

Roasted Broccoli

If you only eat steamed broccoli, then this roasted variety will be a real treat. It doesn't take much more effort, but it takes on a whole new dimension thanks to a hot oven that caramelizes the tender green stems. Serve this alongside any meat or seafood for a delicious and healthy side you'll love.

- 1 pound broccoli florets, trimmed into bite-sized pieces
- 2 tablespoons olive oil
- juice of 1 lemon
- Freshly ground black pepper, to taste

Preheat oven to 400 degrees F.

Lay broccoli on a parchment-lined sheet tray and drizzle with olive oil and lemon juice. Season with freshly ground black pepper.

Bake for 30 minutes, stirring halfway through, until the broccoli is slightly browned and crispy. Serve immediately.

Serves 4

Balsamic Roasted Onions

You may not think of onions as being a side dish, but once you've tried these sweet, delicate morsels, you'll quickly change your mind. Slice the onions with a mandolin to make sure the slices are all equal, ensuring that they'll cook evenly. Use these to top steaks and chops, or even to garnish soups or salads. Once you get creative, you'll find endless uses for them.

- 1 large red onion, sliced thinly
- 1 tablespoon olive oil
- Freshly ground black pepper, to taste
- 1 tablespoon balsamic vinegar

Preheat oven to 400 degrees F.

Lay the sliced onions in a baking dish in a single layer. Drizzle with olive oil. Season with freshly ground black pepper.

Roast for 30 minutes until onions start crisping and browning. Toss cooked onions with the balsamic vinegar and serve.

Serves 4

Paleo Cranberry Sauce

If you're looking for a delicious cranberry sauce to serve alongside your roasted turkey or pork, then look no further than this deliciously tart version. Orange juice and a bit of maple syrup take the place of refined white sugar for a side dish you can enjoy without feeling guilty. Make sure to buy whole oranges and squeeze or juice them yourself for best results.

- 1 pound fresh cranberries
- 1 cup freshly squeezed orange juice
- 1 tablespoon pure maple syrup

Put the cranberries and juice in a saucepan and bring to a boil. Stir every few minutes until the cranberries begin to pop open.

Stir in the maple syrup and cook for a few more minutes. Cool before serving.

Serves 6

Cauliflower Rice

Cauliflower is an amazing vegetable that can take many shapes and forms, and makes an excellent substitute for potatoes, rice, and other starches that are off limits on the Paleo plan. You can use this anywhere you would serve rice. It makes a great addition to stir-fries or alongside fish or chicken. This is a basic version, but like rice, the mild flavor of cauliflower makes it a blank canvas for taking on other flavors. Feel free to experiment until you find something you love.

- ½ head cauliflower
- 1 tablespoon olive or coconut oil
- 2 cloves garlic, minced
- Freshly ground black pepper, to taste

Using a food processor or cheese grater, grate the cauliflower into pieces that are similar to the size of rice granules.

Heat the oil in a medium saucepan over medium heat. Add the garlic and sauté for 1 minute.

Add the cauliflower and cook for 3 to 4 minutes, until cooked through. Season with freshly ground black pepper.

Serve immediately and use anywhere you would use plain rice.

Serves 2

Baked Spaghetti Squash

One ingredient is all it takes for a side dish that will make you swoon. Unlike other winter squash, this variety has a stringy texture that mimics spaghetti. It's amazing when baked and covered in your favorite pasta sauce—you'll never know you're not eating all those carbs. Eat anywhere you would eat pasta, or just eat as a side dish. Either way, we think you'll love it.

- 1 spaghetti squash
- Freshly ground black pepper, to taste

Preheat oven to 400 degrees F.

Remove the stem from the squash and cut in half. Using a very sharp knife will make the process easier.

Put the squash on a baking sheet, season with pepper, and bake for 40 minutes.

Scoop the flesh out, separate it with a fork if necessary, and serve.

Serves 4

Garlicky Wilted Spinach

If you have reservations about eating cooked spinach, they will end with this dish. It's so simple, yet so flavorful, and makes a great, fast and easy side dish to use for practically anything. The best part? It's amazingly good for you as well. While it may seem like this recipe calls for a lot of spinach, it does cook down quite a bit, so don't skimp thinking you have too much.

- 2 tablespoons olive oil
- 2 cloves garlic, minced
- 4 cups baby spinach leaves
- Freshly ground black pepper, to taste

In a large skillet, heat the oil over medium heat. Add the garlic and cook for 2 minutes.

Add the spinach a handful at a time, trying to get it in the pan as quickly as possible. Season with freshly ground black pepper. When spinach is just wilted, remove from heat and be ready to serve, as it is best served as soon as possible.

Serves 2

Quick-Cooked Cabbage

Cabbage is a powerhouse vegetable that is highly underrated and often used as an accent. This quick side dish allows the pungent natural flavors of the cabbage to shine while providing a good dose of fiber, vitamins, and antioxidants. While many cabbage dishes use apples or vinegar to add flavor, this dish is just cabbage, in all its glory—and it's quite tasty.

- 1 tablespoon olive oil
- ¼ head of green cabbage, thinly sliced or grated
- Freshly ground black pepper, to taste

Heat a large skillet over medium-high heat. Add the oil to the skillet, followed by the cabbage. Stir to evenly coat all of the shredded cabbage with the oil. Season with freshly ground black pepper.

Stir and continue cooking for 5 minutes. Serve immediately.

Serves 2

Roasted Baby Carrots

If you've ever been to a five-star restaurant, you may have encountered glazed carrots on the menu, as it is a frequent side dish. While these may be nice, the truth is that carrots have a lot of natural sugar in them, so if you cook them just right, you'll find they are super sweet on their own without any sugary sweet glazes. This recipe proves that, as crunchy baby carrots are roasted to perfection, leaving you with sweet and tender carrots that don't have any added sugar.

- 1 pound baby carrots
- 2 tablespoons olive oil
- Freshly ground black pepper, to taste

Preheat oven to 400 degrees F.

Lay the carrots on a parchment-lined baking sheet in a single layer. Drizzle with olive oil. Season with freshly ground black pepper.

Roast for 30 minutes, or until carrots are lightly browned and fork tender.

Serve immediately.

Serves 4

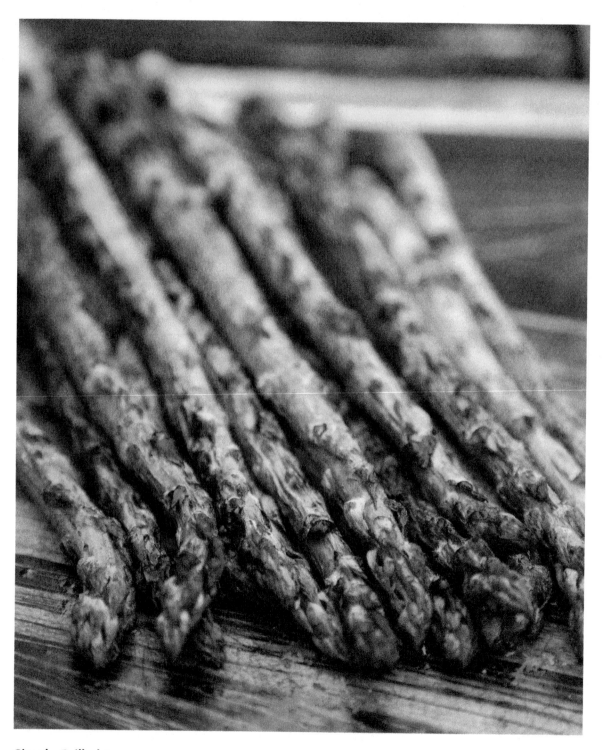

Simple Grilled Asparagus

Simple Grilled Asparagus

Depending on the dish you are serving, sometimes you want a side dish with a lot of competing flavors and textures. Other times, though, you just want something that is good, but that won't outshine your main course. That's the case with this simple grilled asparagus recipe. It's one vegetable, and it's amazing when grilled, but when you serve it alongside a tender steak, it complements rather than takes center stage. It's also easy to make, and will make any meal feel like a special occasion.

- 1 pound asparagus stalks, tough ends trimmed
- 1 tablespoon olive oil
- Freshly ground black pepper, to taste
- Lemon juice, for seasoning

Preheat a gas or charcoal grill to medium-high heat. Toss the asparagus with olive oil and season with freshly ground black pepper and lemon juice.

Lay the asparagus on the grill grates diagonally so that they don't fall through. Cook for 5 to 6 minutes, turning consistently, until they are tender.

Remove from grill and serve immediately.

Serves 4

Paleo Stuffed Zucchini

If you've got a garden, you know that the zucchini patch is a feast or famine situation. The first fruits take their time to appear, but then— watch out! Before long, you'll be overrun with the stuff, and your neighbors will turn the other way when they see you coming. Here's one flavorful way to use excess zucchini. Loaded with garden veggies and homemade sausage, this is Paleo at its best!

- 2 tablespoons olive oil
- ½ cup onion, chopped
- ½ cup red bell pepper, chopped
- ½ cup carrots, chopped
- ½ cup kale, chopped
- 2 tablespoons garlic, minced
- Freshly ground black pepper, to taste
- ½ pound high quality sausage, cooked and crumbled
- ½ cup almond meal
- 1 large egg
- ¼ cup fresh basil, chopped
- 4 small zucchinis

Preheat oven to 400 degrees F. Heat the oil in a large skillet and add the onions, bell pepper, carrots, kale, and garlic. Sauté for 5 minutes, or until tender. Season with freshly ground black pepper.

In a large mixing bowl, combine the sautéed vegetables and the remaining ingredients, except the zucchini. Cut the zucchini lengthwise and scoop out the seeds. Fill the zucchini with the sausage mixture. Cover with aluminum foil and bake for 20 to 30 minutes.

Serves 4

Beef, Celery, Walnut, and Apple Stuffing

Who says stuffing has to be made out of bread? This version is made with lean ground beef, celery, apples, and walnuts, making it amazing and much healthier. The ground beef needs to be very lean so the fat does not change the taste and texture you are looking to create. With the celery, apples, and spices used, the aroma and texture will remain similar to that of traditional stuffing. The result will be much better if you chop your own fresh herbs.

- 1 pound extra-lean, grass-fed ground beef
- 4 stalks celery, diced
- 1 tablespoon olive oil
- 1 apple, diced
- 1 medium onion, diced
- 1 clove garlic, minced
- 2 tablespoons poultry seasoning
- 2 cups walnuts, chopped and toasted
- Freshly ground black pepper, to taste

Preheat oven to 375 degrees F.

Sauté the ground beef and celery with the oil for approximately 3 minutes in a large pan. Be sure to crumble the ground beef into small pieces.

Add the diced apple and onion, and continue to sauté for an additional 2 minutes.

Add the seasoning, minced garlic, and walnuts, and season with freshly ground black pepper to taste. Mix well. The meat should remain somewhat pink, and will finish cooking in the oven.

Place the mixture in a baking dish and cook uncovered for approximately 30 minutes.

Serves 4

Garlic and Herb Mashed Cauliflower

A beautiful substitute for mashed potatoes, this mashed cauliflower side dish is full of flavor as well as loads of vitamins and other good stuff for you. This goes well with meatloaf, Swiss steak, or anything else that you would serve mashed potatoes with—and we bet you won't be able to tell the difference!

- 1 head of cauliflower, washed and cut into florets
- 2 tablespoons olive or coconut oil, divided
- 1 medium sweet onion, chopped
- 3 cloves of garlic, minced
- 1 tablespoon fresh thyme, finely chopped
- 1 tablespoon fresh rosemary, finely chopped
- Freshly ground black pepper, to taste

Steam or boil the cauliflower until soft (about 10 minutes).

Add 1 tablespoon of the oil to a large sauté pan over medium heat. Sauté onion, garlic, and herbs until onion softens and becomes translucent.

Add cauliflower and onion mixture to blender or food processor along with remaining oil. Season with freshly ground black pepper.

Pulse until desired consistency is reached. Serve warm.

Serves 3 to 4

Grilled Tropical Fruit Skewers

If you think fruit can't be a delicious side dish for a savory meal, think again. These easy kebabs go with pork, chicken, and fish, and they even make a nice dessert, especially when sprinkled with a little cinnamon. While the fruit choices in this recipe are delicious, you can use any combination you like. Mangoes, strawberries, and kiwis are all delicious additions depending on what you are serving them with.

- 2 bananas, sliced into bite-sized pieces
- ½ cantaloupe, seeded and cut into bite-sized pieces
- ½ pineapple, cut into bite-sized pieces
- 1 tablespoon coconut oil

Heat a gas or charcoal grill to medium-high. If you're using wooden skewers, soak them for 10 minutes before using.

Skewer the fruit, alternating between types, until you run out.

Brush the fruit with the coconut oil. Lay the skewers on the grill and cook, turning often for about 8 minutes or until edges are lightly charred and fruit is soft.

Serve immediately.

Serves 4

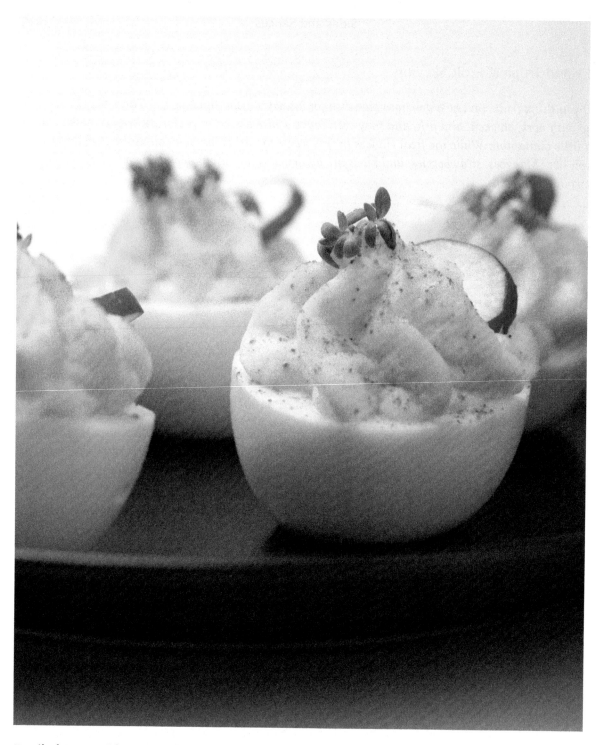

Deviled Eggs with Bacon Bits

Deviled Eggs with Bacon Bits

Deviled eggs are a classic appetizer, but can also be used as a nice side dish for lighter lunches and dinners. They are easy to prepare and universally enjoyed, especially with this recipe that adds bacon bits for a nice, unexpected flavor.

- 6 slices uncured, nitrate-free bacon
- 12 large eggs
- ½ cup olive-oil mayonnaise
- 1 tablespoon mustard
- 1 tablespoon ground cumin
- Freshly ground black pepper, to taste
- Paprika for garnish

Cook bacon in a pan over medium heat until crispy. Let cool and crumble into small bits.

Place eggs in a pot filled with cold water. Bring to a boil for 12 minutes. Remove from the heat, drain, and add cold water immediately to the eggs.

Once the eggs are cool enough to handle, peel and cut in half.

Scoop out the yolks and mash in a bowl with mayonnaise, mustard, cumin, bacon bits, and pepper.

Fill in the cavity of the egg white halves with the yolk, mayonnaise, and bacon filling.

Garnish with paprika or any of your favorite fresh herbs.

Makes 2 dozen

Mango Slaw with Carrots and Red Onion

Coleslaw doesn't need to be boring. This delicious slaw includes bright, tart mangoes and crisp veggies. It goes great with seafood, such as crab cakes, and even lends an interesting twist to a barbecue.

- ½ head of green cabbage, finely shredded
- 1 large carrot, finely grated
- 1 orange or yellow bell pepper, cut into ⅛-inch confetti
- 1 small red onion, thinly sliced
- 1 mango, flesh removed into ⅛-inch-wide matchsticks
- 1 stalk of scallion, finely chopped
- 2 tablespoons olive-oil mayonnaise
- 3 tablespoons white vinegar
- ¼ cup olive oil
- Freshly ground black pepper, to taste

In a large bowl, toss together the cabbage, carrot, bell pepper, onion, mango, and scallions.

In another bowl, mix together the mayonnaise and vinegar. While slowly drizzling in the olive oil, whisk everything together. Season with pepper.

Add the dressing to the vegetables and toss to coat. Refrigerate for at least an hour to allow the flavors to meld.

Serves 4

Cabbage Braised in Duck Fat

Duck fat adds wonderful flavor to everything. In this dish, the savory duck fat braised cabbage is balanced with the sweet tartness of sherry vinegar and apples. If you can't find duck fat, bacon grease is a good alternative.

- 3 tablespoons of duck fat
- 1 medium onion, thinly sliced
- 1 red cabbage, outer wilted leaves and core removed, sliced very thinly
- 1 tablespoon sherry vinegar
- 1 bay leaf
- ½ cup water
- Freshly ground black pepper, to taste
- 1 apple, peeled and grated

Add the duck fat to a large sauté pan over medium-high heat. When the duck fat has melted, add the onion. Sauté the onion until soft and translucent.

Add the cabbage, vinegar, bay leaf, and water to the hot pan. Season with freshly ground black pepper.

Bring the water to a boil and cover. Simmer for about 20 minutes.

Stir in the grated apple and serve.

Serves 4

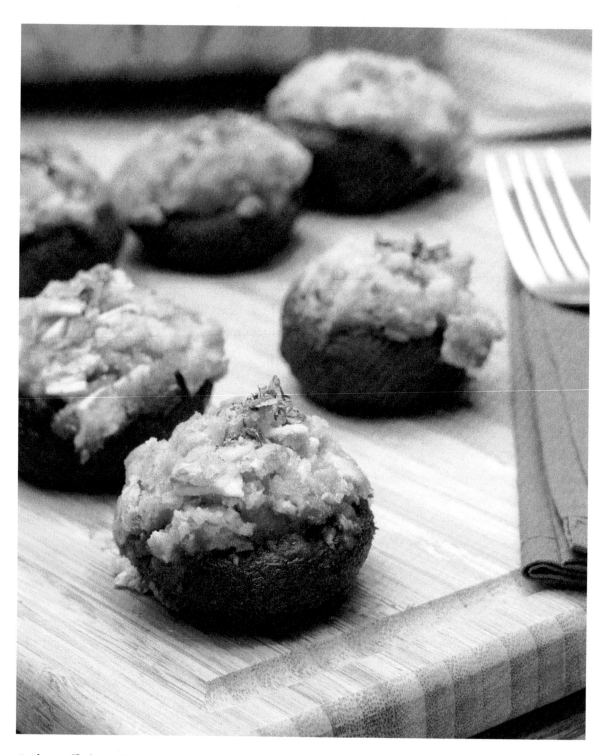

Crab-Stuffed Mushrooms

Crab-Stuffed Mushrooms

Mushrooms can often be forgotten on a Paleo diet, but they are certainly a healthy and tasty addition to any recipe. Mushrooms are often stuffed with cheeses, but these crab-stuffed ones are just as delectable. Simple white button mushrooms are perfect here, but feel free to use any mushroom you have handy that are big enough to stuff.

- 20 button mushrooms, stems and gills removed
- 2 cups crabmeat, cooked and finely chopped
- 3 tablespoons chives, minced

- 3 cloves garlic, minced
- ¼ teaspoon dried oregano
- ¼ teaspoon dried thyme
- ¼ teaspoon mustard
- Freshly ground black pepper, to taste

Preheat oven to 350 degrees F.

Mix all the ingredients except mushrooms together in a bowl. Spoon a generous portion into each mushroom and bake on a baking sheet for about 15 minutes.

Let cool slightly, but serve when still warm.

Serves 2 to 4

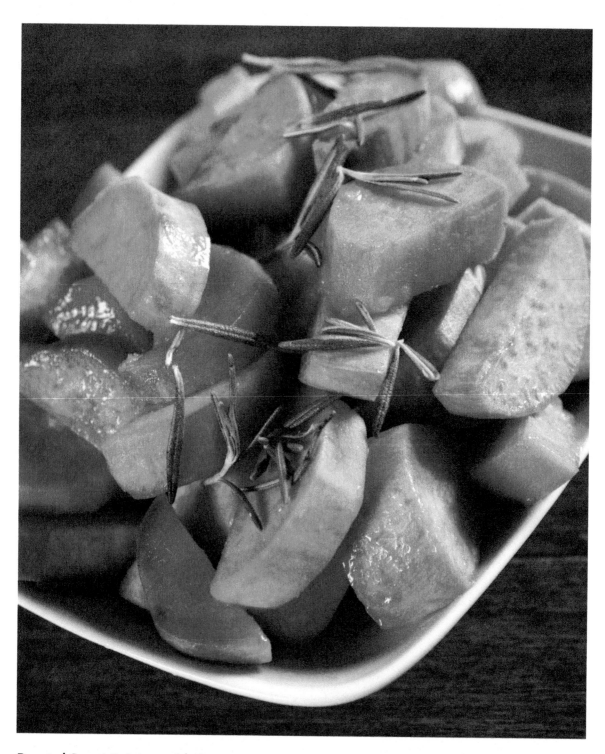

Roasted Sweet Potatoes with Rosemary

Roasted Sweet Potatoes with Rosemary

To make things a little unusual while keeping with the bulkier and orange autumn vegetables, this roasted, cubed, sweet potato dish with a touch of rosemary is perfect for any occasion. Rosemary features strong antioxidant assets, but feel free to use any woody herb such as thyme or sage in place of the rosemary.

- 2 large sweet potatoes, peeled and cut into 1-inch cubes
- 1 large sprig rosemary leaves
- 3 tablespoons olive or coconut oil
- 4 cloves garlic, crushed
- Freshly ground black pepper, to taste

Preheat oven to 425 degrees F.

Fill a pot with cold water, place in the sweet potato cubes, and bring to a rapid boil for 5 minutes. Quickly drain the potatoes in a colander and let steam and dry.

Using a mortar and pestle, grind the rosemary leaves.

Heat a roasting pan on the stove over medium-low heat, add the oil, rosemary, and sweet potato cubes and season with pepper. Stir until all ingredients are blended and hot.

Place the roasting pan in the oven and roast for approximately 20 to 25 minutes or until crispy and tender. Be sure to stir the potatoes occasionally for an even texture.

Serve warm.

Serves 2 to 4

Tender and Flavorful Herb-Laced Carrots

Orange vegetables are always a hit around Thanksgiving and fall. Despite the simplicity of this side dish, it is delicious and extremely easy to prepare, and will add a nice touch to any dinner.

- 3 cloves garlic, minced
- Juice and zest of 1 orange
- Handful of fresh parsley leaves, chopped
- 2 tablespoons olive or coconut oil
- 2 large carrots, thinly sliced
- Freshly ground black pepper, to taste
- 1 cup chicken stock

Preheat oven to 350 degrees F.

Combine the garlic, orange zest, and parsley. Chop together until fine. Rub the baking dish with one half of the oil and dust with some of the garlic, zest, and parsley mixture.

Line the bottom of the dish with carrot slices, brush with the rest of the oil and season lightly with pepper. Sprinkle some more of the garlic, zest, and parsley mixture.

Repeat while layering carrot slices. Top with orange juice and just enough chicken stock to cover. Line with wax paper on top of the carrots to prevent them from drying out.

Place in the hot oven and bake for approximately 20 to 25 minutes or until carrots are very tender.

Serves 2

Sweet Potato Salad

Sweet potatoes, pineapple, and toasted pecans create this delightful side dish that is sweet and flavorful. The pecans, celery, and bell pepper add a nice crunch to the dish, as well as some good nutrition.

- 2 pounds sweet potatoes
- ¼ cup olive-oil mayonnaise
- 1 tablespoon mustard
- 4 celery stalks, chopped
- 1 small red bell pepper, diced
- 1 cup fresh pineapple, diced
- 2 scallions, finely chopped
- Freshly ground black pepper, to taste
- ½ cup toasted pecans, coarsely chopped
- Fresh chives, chopped, to taste

Preheat oven to 400 degrees F. Roast sweet potatoes on oven rack for one hour. Remove and let stand until cool enough to handle. Peel sweet potatoes and cut into ¾-inch cubes.

Whisk together the mayonnaise and mustard in a large bowl.

Add the sweet potatoes, celery, bell pepper, pineapple, and scallions. Mix well and season with pepper. Cover and chill for 1 hour.

Stir in the pecans just before serving and garnish with the chives.

Serves 4

Whipped Carrot Soufflé

This dish is reminiscent of sweet potato casserole at Thanksgiving time, only without the marshmallows. A bit of spice, a bit of sweetness—this carrot dish makes a nice accompaniment to almost any meat.

- 1 quart chicken broth
- 2 pounds baby carrots
- 3 large eggs
- 2 tablespoons onion, minced
- ½ cup coconut oil, melted
- 1 tablespoon coconut flour
- 2 teaspoons fresh lemon juice
- ¼ teaspoon cinnamon
- ¼ cup pure maple syrup
- Freshly ground black pepper, to taste

Preheat oven to 350 degrees F.

Add the chicken broth to a pot and bring to a simmer. Add the carrots and cook until tender.

Put the carrots into a mixing bowl and beat until smooth.

Mix in the eggs, onion, coconut oil, coconut flour, lemon juice, cinnamon, and maple syrup. Beat the mixture until very smooth. Season with freshly ground black pepper.

Scoop the mix into a large casserole dish and place in oven. Bake in oven for 45 minutes until top is lightly browned. Serve warm.

Serves 4

Crispy Lemon Green Beans

Lemon adds a touch of acidity that brings out the great flavor of fresh green beans. Roasting the beans in the oven makes them crispy and gives them an unexpected crunch you'll love.

- 1 pound of fresh green beans
- 2 tablespoons olive or coconut oil
- 2 teaspoons of dried rosemary
- 2 teaspoons of dried sage
- Freshly ground black pepper, to taste
- 1 lemon, thinly sliced, seeds removed

Preheat oven to 400 degrees F.

Add washed and trimmed green beans to a casserole dish. Pour oil over top of beans.

Sprinkle rosemary and sage, and mix ingredients until well coated. Season with freshly ground black pepper.

Place the lemon slices in an even layer over the green beans. Bake for 30 to 35 minutes until they are crispy.

Serves 4

Brussels Sprouts with Hazelnuts

This is a very simple way to roast Brussels sprouts, leaving them tender and full of flavor. Watch the hazelnuts carefully in the oven so they don't burn.

- 3 tablespoons olive or coconut oil
- 1 pound Brussels sprouts, trimmed and halved or quartered, depending on size
- ¼ cup hazelnuts, chopped
- Freshly ground black pepper, to taste

Preheat oven to 450 degrees F.

Toss the Brussels sprouts and hazelnuts with the oil and put onto a cookie sheet.

Sprinkle with pepper and place sheet into oven.

Bake for 15 minutes, occasionally turning the Brussels sprouts with a wooden spoon.

Serves 4

Kale with Walnuts and Cranberries

Kale is a good source of protein and vitamins. Cranberries and walnuts add excellent flavor to this side dish that goes great with beef or chicken. If you can find cranberries that have no added sugar, you should get those; otherwise, use dried tart cherries.

- 1 pound bunch of kale with tough stems removed, washed and torn into large pieces
- 2 tablespoons olive oil
- ½ medium red onion, finely chopped
- 3 cloves garlic, minced
- ½ cup walnuts, chopped
- ¼ cup dried cranberries, preferably with no added sugar
- Freshly ground black pepper, to taste

Bring a large of pot of water to a boil. Add the kale and cook until tender and bright green, about 4 or 5 minutes. Remove the kale and run under cold water to cool.

In a large sauté pan, add the oil over medium heat. Add the onion and sauté until soft.

Stir in the garlic and walnuts and cook until the nuts are golden, about 2 minutes. Mix the cranberries in, and then add the kale.

Toss gently with the onion/cranberry mixture. Season with pepper and serve warm.

Serves 2

Acorn Squash and Yams Cooked in Duck Fat

Duck fat is a great way to roast squash and root vegetables. The heated fat creates a nice crispy texture and also adds some amazing flavor to the dish.

- 1 small acorn squash, thinly sliced
- 1 large yam, peeled and thinly sliced into coins
- 2 large parsnips, peeled and cut into batons
- 5 whole garlic cloves
- 2 tablespoons duck fat, melted
- 1 tablespoon dried thyme
- 1 tablespoon dried rosemary, crushed
- Freshly ground black pepper, to taste

Preheat oven to 400 degrees F.

Add all of the ingredients in a large bowl and toss well to coat evenly. Spread the mixture out onto a baking sheet.

Roast in oven 30 to 40 minutes until vegetables are soft. Transfer to a large platter and serve warm.

Serves 4

Roasted Baby Artichokes

Baby artichokes are a treat because almost the entire thing is edible. The flavor of artichoke is subtle and delicious and doesn't need much improvement. This is a simple way of roasting the artichokes that brings out the best flavor.

- 1 lemon, halved
- 10 baby artichokes
- 2 tablespoons olive oil
- 2 cloves garlic, minced
- Freshly ground black pepper, to taste

Preheat oven to 400 degrees F.

Fill a bowl with cold water and squeeze the lemon over the bowl.

Cut about a quarter off the end of each artichoke (opposite the stem). Remove all the hard outer leaves. Use a paring knife to remove the remaining hard skin near the base of the artichoke.

Cut each baby artichoke in half lengthwise and toss in the lemon water. When done cutting all of the artichokes, drain the water and pat dry with a paper towel.

Toss the artichokes with oil, garlic, and a little pepper.

Spread the artichokes out in an even layer onto a baking sheet. Roast for 25 to 30 minutes until soft. Serve warm with sliced lemon.

Serves 2

Roast Turnips with Bacon and Apples

Bacon is loaded with protein and fat and pairs beautifully with roasted root vegetables like turnips. The paprika in this dish adds a bit of smokiness that is very pleasant.

- 4 turnips, ends removed and chopped into bite-sized pieces
- 2 Granny Smith apples, peeled, cored, seeded, and sliced ½-inch thick
- 2 tablespoons bacon grease, melted
- 1 teaspoon smoked paprika
- 1 teaspoon garlic powder
- Freshly ground black pepper, to taste
- 2 strips of uncured, nitrate-free, thick-cut bacon, cooked and crumbled, to garnish

Preheat oven to 400 degrees F.

In a large bowl, toss the turnips and apples with the bacon grease, paprika, garlic powder, and pepper.

Transfer mixture to a large casserole dish. Bake uncovered for 20 minutes, stirring occasionally.

Turn oven down to 350 degrees F and continue to bake for another 20 minutes or until the turnips are soft.

Remove from oven and sprinkle the bacon over the top.

Serves 3 to 4

Braised Cabbage and Bacon

This is a straightforward and luscious side to any turkey or beef entrée, and the bacon adds a flavorful element to the braised cabbage. This recipe can replace any of your usual green vegetable sides. The key to fast preparation is to have a very finely chopped cabbage to allow for a faster cooking time.

- 2 cups chicken stock
- 6 slices uncured, nitrate-free bacon, chopped
- Small handful of thyme leaves
- 1 medium green cabbage, finely sliced
- Freshly ground black pepper, to taste
- 4 tablespoons olive or coconut oil

Bring the stock, bacon, and thyme leaves to a boil in a large pot. Add the cabbage, boil for 5 minutes and then reduce to a simmer.

Simmer the cabbage until just tender to your taste. Season with freshly ground black pepper.

Add some stock during the simmering process if you feel it has reduced too much.

Add the oil, season to taste, and serve immediately.

Serves 2 to 4

Sweet Potato Mash with Pecans

Mashed sweet potatoes are very easy to prepare and do not require ingredients that you probably don't already have, which is always a plus. When eaten by themselves, sweet potatoes can be quite sweet. However, the green onions add a bite, and the pecans give a terrific nutty taste and add a nice, crunchy texture.

- 3 large sweet potatoes, peeled and cubed
- ½ cup olive or coconut oil
- Freshly ground black pepper, to taste
- 2 green onions, chopped
- ⅛ teaspoon ground cinnamon
- ¼ cup toasted pecans, chopped

Boil potatoes in large pot until soft enough to mash.

Strain the potatoes and put them back in the pot. Add the oil and mash until potatoes are smooth and silky. Season with freshly ground black pepper.

Add onions with the cinnamon and mix completely to ensure the cinnamon is dispersed consistently. Add the pecans.

Serve warm.

Serves 4

Creamy Tomato Baked Scallops

Scallops can be prepared in a variety of ways, though they are typically pan-fried. When the weather permits, they can also easily be grilled. However you decide to cook them, they are easy to prepare and require very minimal time. Scallops, as nutritious as they are, can be bland, so adding flavors to them is a good idea. This recipe accomplishes this with the help of a delectable and rich tomato sauce, added coconut milk, and fresh oregano.

- 1 tablespoon coconut oil
- 1 cup red onion, chopped
- 3 cloves garlic, minced
- ¼ cup coconut milk
- ¼ cup tomato sauce
- Fresh oregano, finely chopped, to taste
- Freshly ground black pepper, to taste
- 12 medium scallops
- 2 medium tomatoes, seeded and diced

Preheat oven to 475 degrees F.

Over medium-high heat, sauté the onions and the coconut oil in a medium skillet. Cook for several minutes, or until the onion becomes slightly softened.

Add the minced garlic and cook on medium-low heat.

Sauté for a few minutes before adding the coconut milk and tomato sauce, and follow up with the oregano. Season to taste with pepper. Mix well and cook for approximately 2 to 3 more minutes.

Place the scallops on the bottom of a baking dish that is large enough to keep them from overlapping each other. Distribute the coconut milk and tomato mixture on top of the scallops and make sure they are all well coated. Finish by sprinkling the diced tomatoes over the scallops and bake uncovered for approximately 15 to 20 minutes. Serve warm.

Serves 4

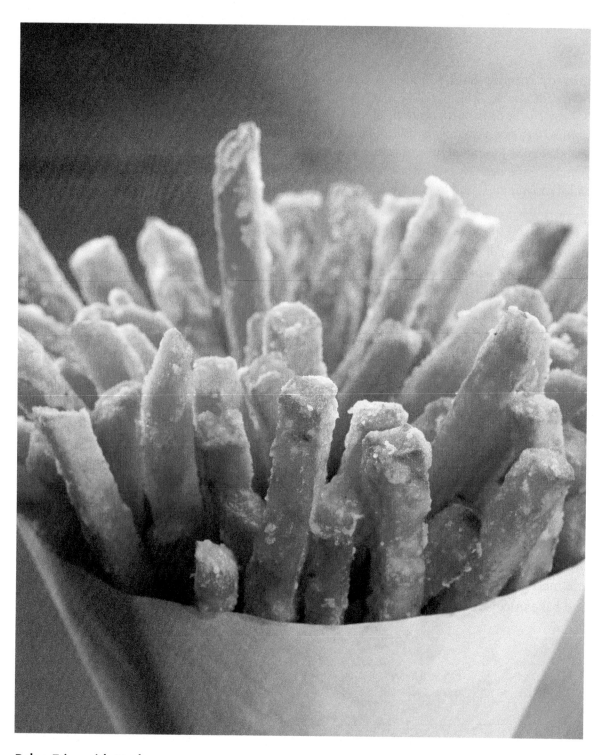

Paleo Fries with Herbs

Paleo Fries with Herbs

Great with chicken drumsticks or thighs, nothing can beat these fries. The natural flavors from the herbs offer a mouthwatering combination, and the fries act as a great way to soak up any sauces on your plate from your chicken.

- 1½ teaspoons oregano, finely chopped
- 1½ teaspoons parsley, finely chopped
- ½ teaspoon thyme, finely chopped
- 4 large sweet potatoes, peeled and cut into evenly sized strips
- 1½ teaspoons ground pepper
- 2 tablespoons coconut oil, melted

Preheat oven to 425 degrees F. Place the oven rack in the middle position.

Combine all of the herbs, pepper, and sweet potatoes in a gallon-size freezer bag. Toss well to disperse the herbs evenly and then add the coconut oil.

Lay potatoes on a baking sheet in an even layer. Sprinkle the herb mixture on top.

Bake for 25 minutes, and then flip the potatoes around to cook for approximately another 15 to 20 minutes.

Serve hot.

Serves 4

Stovetop Spiced Nuts

Nuts as a side dish? The nutrients—especially protein—contained in this mixture of nuts make it the perfect side to any lunch or light dinner entrée. The mixture of herbs will add a nice touch, and you can make these in bulk to have them readily available for your lunch box. These are also a great addition to salads to add a nice crunch.

- ⅔ cup whole almonds
- ⅔ cup whole pecans
- ⅔ cup whole hazelnuts

- 1 teaspoon chili powder
- ½ teaspoon cumin
- 1 tablespoon coconut oil, melted

Toast all of the nuts in a large skillet over medium-high heat. This will only take a few minutes and will not require any butter.

Combine the spices in a small bowl. Mix well to ensure an even consistency.

When the nuts have completely toasted and taken on a golden brown tone, remove from heat and drizzle them with the oil. Make sure the nuts are coated well. Sprinkle with the spice mixture.

Serves 4 to 6

Bacon and Kale

Roasted kale becomes thin, crispy, and smoky, making it a wonderful accompaniment for bacon. It only takes 2 to 3 minutes to cook, though, so watch it closely.

- 1 pound kale
- 1 tablespoon olive oil

- 6 slices uncured, nitrate-free bacon, cooked and crumbled
- Freshly ground black pepper, to taste

Preheat oven to 375 degrees F. Wash the kale carefully and cut it into 2-inch pieces, discarding the stems. Toss the kale with the olive oil on a large cookie sheet.

Roast the kale for 2 to 3 minutes, or until it starts to become crisp. Transfer it to a serving bowl and toss it with the bacon and pepper.

Serves 4

Tex-Mex Coleslaw

This light salad is the perfect meal for a warm summer night. Crisp and refreshing, it provides a healthy dose of protein and just the right crunch! Serve at a barbecue for a classic combination that will never fail you!

- 1 cup chicken, cooked and shredded
- 1 cup cabbage, shredded
- ½ cup red bell pepper, diced
- 1 green onion, chopped
- 1 small tomato, diced
- ½ cup fresh cilantro, chopped
- ¼ cup olive oil
- 3 tablespoons lime juice
- ½ teaspoon cumin
- Freshly ground black pepper, to taste

Combine the chicken, cabbage, bell pepper, onion, and tomato in a medium bowl.

In another bowl, whisk together the remaining ingredients to make a dressing. Pour the dressing over the salad and toss gently. Refrigerate for up to 4 hours before serving to meld flavors.

Serves 4

Paleo Barbecue Sauce

Most store-bought barbecue sauces are going to be loaded with sugar, even if they don't taste particularly sweet. This homemade version is spicy and complex—perfect for slow-cooked meats, grilled chicken, or anywhere else you would use barbecue sauce.

- 1 tablespoon olive or coconut oil
- 2 cloves garlic, minced
- 2 shallots, minced
- 1 teaspoon spicy brown mustard
- 1 teaspoon smoked paprika
- 1 teaspoon chili powder
- 1 teaspoon ground cumin
- 1 cup chicken broth
- Juice of 1 lime
- 1 (6-ounce) can tomato paste
- Freshly ground black pepper, to taste

In a medium saucepan, heat the oil over medium heat. Add the shallots and garlic. Cook until soft, about 3 minutes.

Add the mustard and spices and continue to cook, stirring for 1 more minute.

Add the broth, lime juice, and tomato paste and bring to a boil. Season with freshly ground black pepper.

Reduce to a simmer and cook for about 45 minutes. Allow to cool. For a smooth sauce, puree in a blender or food processor.

Makes 2 cups

Dill Seafood Sauce

This easy-to-use sauce is a delicious addition to crab cakes, shrimp, or just about any kind of seafood. It's also a great dip for veggies at a party, and it goes great with hot wings, too.

- 1 large egg
- Juice of 1 lemon
- 1 cup olive oil
- 1 tablespoon dried dill
- 1 teaspoon garlic powder
- 1 teaspoon onion powder
- Freshly ground black pepper, to taste

Put the egg and lemon juice in a food processor or blender. Turn it on and slowly stream in the oil.

Add the spices and continue blending until smooth and creamy. Season with freshly ground black pepper. Chill before serving.

Makes 1 cup

Easy Garlic Butter Sauce

This sauce is easy to make and makes plain chicken breasts or vegetables perk up instantly. Store leftovers in the refrigerator and warm a little in the microwave if necessary.

- ¼ cup olive or coconut oil
- 2 cloves garlic, minced
- Freshly ground black pepper, to taste
- 1 tablespoon finely chopped fresh parsley

Heat a small saucepan over medium heat. Add the oil. Add the garlic and cook for about 2 minutes, until it starts to turn brown. Remove from heat.

Season with freshly ground black pepper. Stir in the parsley and serve.

Makes ¼ cup

Rosemary Aioli

Aioli is just a fancy name for mayonnaise with garlic added to it. While it's a rich and delicious combination on its own, this version gets a bright kick from the addition of fresh chopped rosemary. In this recipe, you'll make the mayo from scratch, but if you're in a hurry you can just blend the garlic and rosemary with a prepared olive-oil version. This is delicious with baked chicken or roasted vegetables.

- 1 large egg
- Juice of 1 lemon
- ¼ teaspoon ground mustard powder
- 1 cup olive oil
- 2 cloves garlic, minced
- 1 tablespoon fresh rosemary, chopped

Put the egg, lemon juice, and mustard powder in a blender or food processor. Slowly drizzle in the oil and blend until creamy. Add the garlic and rosemary and continue blending until smooth. Chill before serving.

Makes 1 cup

Cocktail Sauce

Cocktail sauce is one of those things most people buy in a jar, but it's actually pretty easy to make at home—no cooking necessary! The end result is much less expensive and better for you than any bottled version. Use this for shrimp cocktail or anywhere else you have the need for this spicy tomato-based dipping sauce.

- 1 (6-ounce) can tomato paste
- 4 tablespoons horseradish
- Juice of 1 small lemon

Combine all ingredients in a small bowl and mix thoroughly. Chill before serving, if desired.

Makes ½ cup

Homemade Buffalo Sauce

While this is more effort than simply grabbing a bottle at the store, once you taste a bite of this spicy sauce on your wings, eggs, or appetizers, you'll immediately notice the difference. While many bottled versions are simply just hot, this homemade version has some heat, but with a much more complex and interesting flavor.

- 10 Fresno chilies
- ½ teaspoon olive or coconut oil
- ½ small onion, chopped
- 3 cloves garlic, minced
- Freshly ground black pepper, to taste
- 3 cups water, divided
- 1 cup apple cider vinegar

Stem and seed the chilies. Slice and set aside.

Heat a small saucepan over medium heat and add the oil. When heated, add the onion, garlic, and chilies. Season with freshly ground black pepper.

Add 2 cups water and bring to a boil. Boil for about 10 minutes, stirring occasionally.

Add 1 more cup water and turn the heat down to medium. Cook until the water is evaporated and the peppers are soft.

In a blender or food processor, add the chilies, onion, and garlic and blend until smooth. Slowly add in the vinegar while continuing to blend until smooth.

Makes 1½ cups

Mango Chutney

This is a yummy dish that works well with grilled fish or chicken, and it goes wonderfully with crab cakes as well. Sweet and savory, you'll enjoy this with a variety of dishes. Make sure your mangoes are ripe before trying this recipe, otherwise you won't get the full flavor.

- 1 tablespoon coconut oil
- 1 garlic clove, minced
- 1 tablespoon fresh ginger, chopped
- ½ small red onion, minced
- 1 red bell pepper, chopped
- 2 ripe mangoes, pitted and chopped
- Juice of 1 lime
- 1 tablespoon curry powder
- 1 teaspoon red pepper flakes
- Freshly ground black pepper, to taste

In a small saucepan, heat the coconut oil over medium heat. Add the garlic and ginger and sauté for 2 minutes.

Add the onion and bell pepper and cook for 2 more minutes.

Add the rest of the ingredients and continue cooking until softened, about 5 more minutes.

Simmer about 10 minutes. Serve.

Makes 3 cups

Homemade Nut Butter

You can use whatever nuts you want here—almonds, pecans, cashews, and walnuts all work well. This is a great alternative to store-bought versions that contain added oils, refined sugar, and other ingredients you just don't need in your diet. Enjoy this with celery or apples for a crunchy and healthy snack.

- 2 cups raw nuts of your choice
- ¼ cup macadamia nut oil

Put the nuts in a food processor and process until finely ground. Stream in the oil and continue pureeing until you have a butter-like texture. Refrigerate any leftovers.

Makes about 2 cups

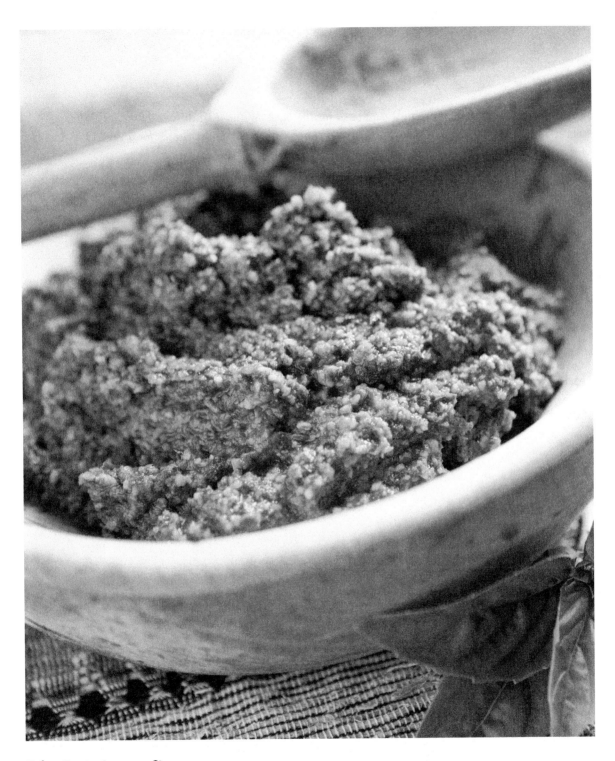

Paleo Pesto (page 278)

Paleo Pesto

Pesto is a popular Italian sauce that uses basil for the base. While it traditionally includes cheese, this version skips it. We don't think you'll miss it though. Try using other herbs for a variety of flavors. Mint and cilantro work especially well.

- 2 cups packed fresh basil leaves
- ½ cup walnuts
- ½ cup olive oil
- Juice of 1 lemon
- Freshly ground black pepper, to taste

Put the basil in a food processor and pulse until well chopped. Add the walnuts and continue chopping.

Slowly stream in the olive oil and lemon juice and puree until you have a smooth sauce. Season with freshly ground black pepper.

Refrigerate any leftover sauce.

Makes 2 cups

9

VEGETABLES AND VEGAN DISHES

Paleo Stuffed Tomatoes

Tomatoes are the glory of the summer garden—robust, sweet, and fragrant. Grow them yourself or buy locally grown tomatoes at a farmer's market. Store them at room temperature for up to five days, and don't refrigerate them, as this destroys their delicate taste. Make this quick and easy dish for a light Paleo lunch, or serve it with tuna salad.

- 2 tablespoons olive or coconut oil
- ½ cup mushrooms, chopped
- ½ cup shallots or leeks, chopped
- ½ cup baby spinach, chopped
- Freshly ground black pepper, to taste
- ½ cup walnuts, chopped
- 4 large beefsteak tomatoes, cored

Preheat oven to 400 degrees F. Heat the oil in a saucepan. Add the vegetables (not the tomatoes) and sauté for 5 minutes, or until tender. Season with freshly ground black pepper. Add the walnuts.

Fill the tomatoes with the veggie mixture and place them on a baking sheet. Bake for 15 to 25 minutes, or until tender and the skins are beginning to crack.

Serves 4

Sweet Potato Salad

This dish contains sweet potatoes, pecans, and dried fruit, and will leave you feeling full without the addition of meat. Serve this dish with steamed greens or a salad for a complete meal.

- ¼ cup olive oil
- Juice and zest of 2 limes
- 2 tablespoons pure maple syrup
- 1 teaspoon fresh ginger, grated
- 1 teaspoon curry powder
- 2 large sweet potatoes, peeled, cubed and steamed until tender
- ½ cup pecans, chopped
- ¼ cup cilantro, chopped
- ¼ cup onion, chopped
- ¼ cup dried cherries
- Freshly ground black pepper, to taste

Combine the oil, lime juice and zest, syrup, ginger, and curry powder in a bowl.

Toss the sweet potatoes, pecans, cilantro, onions, and cherries lightly together in another bowl. Add the dressing and toss again. Season with freshly ground black pepper.

Serve at room temperature.

Serves 4

Paleo Ratatouille

Ratatouille is the perfect vegetarian dinner for a warm, summer evening. Roast the season's bounty to bring out the flavors of the vegetables. Eggplant has a meaty texture and will fill you up without the addition of meat. Choose the freshest vegetables you can find—preferably from your own garden.

- 2 cups eggplant, cubed
- 1 red onion, peeled and slivered
- 3 carrots, peeled and sliced
- 1 cup zucchini rounds
- 1 large green bell pepper, sliced
- 1 large red bell pepper, sliced
- 1 cup summer squash rounds
- 2 fresh plum tomatoes, seeded and quartered
- Freshly ground black pepper, to taste
- 2 tablespoons olive oil
- 1 teaspoon garlic, minced
- 1 teaspoon thyme
- ½ teaspoon marjoram

Preheat oven to 425 degrees F. Spread the vegetables out on a large baking sheet. Season with freshly ground black pepper.

Mix the olive oil, garlic and herbs in a bowl. Drizzle over the vegetables and stir to coat them.

Roast for 15 to 20 minutes, until the vegetables are tender and glistening.

Serves 4

Grilled Pineapple and Sweet Potatoes

When you're craving potatoes, try sweet potatoes instead. They're high in carotene and fiber, and lower in sugar and starch than white potatoes. They pair beautifully with pineapple on the grill for a sweet and smoky dish.

- 2 large sweet potatoes, peeled and cut in cubes
- 1 pineapple, cored and cut in cubes
- 2 tablespoons olive or coconut oil
- 1 tablespoon honey
- 1 teaspoon cinnamon
- Freshly ground black pepper, to taste

Preheat the grill. Place the sweet potatoes on a microwave-safe dish. Cover them and microwave for 8 minutes. Sweet potatoes take a long time to cook, but microwaving them first accelerates the process.

Spray a grill basket with cooking spray. Place the sweet potatoes in the grill basket and grill them for 8 to 10 minutes, stirring frequently, until tender. Add the pineapple and grill an additional 3 to 5 minutes.

Mix the oil, honey, and cinnamon in a bowl and pour over the pineapple and sweet potatoes. Stir to combine, cook for one more minute, and remove from the heat.

Serves 4

Winter Veggie Stew

This hearty stew is vegan, but it's also very filling. Many people are surprised to find that a lot of vegan dishes fit on the Paleo plan, and that it is quite possible to not eat meat and get a lot protein. Leafy greens, such as the kale and spinach in this dish, are loaded with fiber and protein, as well as vitamins and minerals that will keep your body going all day long.

- 2 tablespoons olive oil
- 1 small onion, minced
- 2 cloves garlic, minced
- 2 carrots, sliced
- 1 cup mushrooms, sliced
- 1 stalk celery, chopped
- 1 tablespoon Italian seasoning
- 4 cups packed baby spinach
- 1 large bunch Tuscan kale, chopped
- Freshly ground black pepper, to taste
- 6 cups vegetable broth
- 1 (15-ounce) can of chopped tomatoes

Heat the oil in a large soup pot or Dutch oven over medium heat. Add the onions, garlic, carrots, mushrooms, and celery and cook for 10 minutes until veggies are soft.

Add the Italian season, spinach, and kale and stir until everything is combined. Season with freshly ground black pepper.

Add the vegetable broth and tomatoes with juices. Bring to a boil. Reduce heat and simmer for 20 minutes until carrots are soft. Serve immediately.

Serves 4

Baked Southwestern Sweet Potato

Sweet potatoes are a great alternative to white potatoes on the Paleo diet, as they are loaded with fiber, vitamins, and minerals and have significantly less starch. While you don't want to eat unlimited amounts, they are perfectly fine and even healthy when eaten once in a while, as with this easy and flavorful dish that can be a meal in itself.

- 1 medium sweet potato
- 1 teaspoon cumin
- 1 teaspoon chili powder
- Freshly ground black pepper, to taste
- 2 tablespoons prepared tomato salsa
- Fresh cilantro, chopped, for garnish

Preheat oven to 400 degrees F. Put sweet potato directly on the rack in the oven.

Bake for 30 minutes, remove from the oven, and prick all over with a fork. Return to the oven and bake for 30 more minutes. Remove from the oven and allow to cool for 5 minutes.

Cut open the top and remove the flesh from the skin. Put flesh in a bowl and mash with the cumin and chili powder. Season with freshly ground black pepper.

Top with the salsa and cilantro and serve.

Serves 1

Italian Spiced "Pasta"

This dish is loaded with vegetables. In fact, it is pretty much nothing but! The zucchini, when sliced with a mandolin, makes an excellent substitute for pasta that is both filling and high in fiber, but without all those pesky carbs. Serve this with a green salad for a delicious plant-based meal you'll return to again and again.

- 2 tablespoons olive oil
- 1 small onion, diced
- 1 red bell pepper, diced
- 1 cup broccoli florets
- ½ small eggplant, peeled and diced
- Freshly ground black pepper, to taste
- 2 large zucchini
- 1 tablespoon Italian seasoning
- 2 tablespoons pine nuts, toasted
- Fresh chopped basil, for garnish

Heat the oil in a large skillet over medium-high heat. Add all of the vegetables but the zucchini and cook until soft, about 12 minutes. Season with freshly ground black pepper.

Bring a large pot of water to a boil. Slice the zucchini into thin slices of pasta using a mandolin or sharp knife.

Add the zucchini to the boiling water and cook for 3 minutes or until soft and noodle-like.

To serve, put a mound of zucchini on a plate and top with the cooked vegetable mixture. Garnish with the Italian seasoning, pine nuts, and basil.

Serves 4

Peanut and Sweet Potato Stew

Adapted for the Paleo diet, this flavorful dish is still as filling as possible thanks to the addition of extra veggies, along with the hearty sweet potatoes. This warmly spiced dish is best served on a chilly winter night when you're looking for something comforting, but also healthy.

- 2 tablespoons olive oil
- 1 medium onion, chopped
- 2 fresh jalapeños, seeded and minced
- 2 teaspoons fresh ginger, minced
- 2 cloves garlic, minced
- 2 teaspoons ground cumin
- ¼ teaspoon ground cinnamon
- ⅛ teaspoon crushed red pepper
- ¼ teaspoon ground coriander
- Freshly ground black pepper, to taste
- 2 large sweet potatoes, peeled and cubed
- 1 (28-ounce) can diced tomatoes
- 1 pound fresh green beans, trimmed and cut into bite-sized pieces
- 2 cups vegetable broth
- ¼ cup natural peanut butter, no oils or sugar added

In a large Dutch oven or soup pot, heat the oil over medium heat. Add the onions, jalapeño peppers, ginger, garlic, and spices and cook for 5 minutes. Season with freshly ground black pepper.

Add the sweet potatoes and cook for 5 minutes more.

Add the tomatoes, green beans, and vegetable broth and bring to a boil. Reduce heat and simmer for 20 minutes, or until sweet potatoes are tender when pierced with a fork.

Stir in the peanut butter and simmer until heated through. Serve immediately.

Serves 4

Baked Eggplant Steaks with Quick Tomato Sauce

Eggplant is a great vegetarian alternative to meat as it has a hearty, firm texture that holds up well to many cooking methods. This version has thick-cut slices topped with a zesty tomato sauce. The addition of fennel seed will give a spicy flavor reminiscent of Italian cooking.

- 1 (28-ounce) can crushed tomatoes
- 1 tablespoon fennel seeds
- 1 tablespoon Italian seasoning
- Freshly ground black pepper, to taste
- 2 tablespoons olive oil
- 1 large eggplant, peeled and cut into 1-inch-thick slices
- 1 tablespoon balsamic vinegar
- Fresh basil, chopped, for garnish

In a large saucepan, add the crushed tomatoes, fennel, and Italian seasoning. Season with freshly ground black pepper. Bring to a simmer and cook on low while you cook the eggplant.

Heat a large skillet over medium-high heat and add the olive oil. Add the eggplant slices and cook until browned on both sides and eggplant is tender when pierced with a fork.

Stir the balsamic vinegar into the sauce.

To serve, put the eggplant steaks on plates and top with the tomato sauce. Garnish with fresh chopped basil.

Serves 4

Sweet Potato and Leek Casserole

This easy dish gets its mild and sweet flavor from sautéed leeks and thinly sliced sweet potatoes that are baked in harmony until tender. This dish works well as either a side dish or a main course if served with a salad, and is an impressive take on what is normally a sugary sweet Thanksgiving side dish.

- 2 tablespoons olive oil
- 2 leeks, white parts only, sliced
- 2 cloves garlic, minced
- 1 tablespoon fresh rosemary, chopped
- Freshly ground black pepper, to taste
- 2 large sweet potatoes, peeled and thinly sliced
- ¼ cup vegetable broth

Preheat oven to 400 degrees F.

Heat the oil in a large skillet. Add the leeks, garlic, and rosemary and sauté until leeks are soft, about 8 minutes. Season with freshly ground black pepper.

In an 8 x 8-inch casserole dish, cover the bottom with an even layer of sweet potatoes. Top with some of the leeks, and continue layering the leeks and potatoes until you reach the top of the pan or both are gone.

Drizzle with the vegetable broth. Cover with foil and bake for 45 minutes. Serve immediately.

Serves 4

Steamed Artichokes and Tomatoes Over Cauliflower "Rice"

As you probably know by now, rice is strictly forbidden on the Paleo diet, which can make it difficult to find vegetarian dishes that fit the bill. This dish is simply a mixture of steamed vegetables, but the way the cauliflower is chopped makes it seem like you are eating rice. It's a unique twist that is also a healthy option.

- 1 head of cauliflower
- 2 tablespoons olive oil
- 1 tablespoon Italian seasoning
- ½ cup water
- 1 package frozen artichoke hearts, thawed
- 1 pint cherry tomatoes
- ½ cup sun-dried tomatoes, chopped
- Freshly ground black pepper, to taste
- 2 tablespoons toasted pine nuts
- Fresh basil, chopped, for garnish

Cut the cauliflower into florets. Using a food processor, chop the cauliflower into pieces that resemble rice. Chop in batches if necessary, being careful not to puree. It's okay if they are slightly larger than raw rice, but try to get them as small as possible.

Heat the oil in a medium saucepan and add the cauliflower. Stir to coat.

Add the Italian seasoning and ½ cup water and stir.

Put the artichoke hearts, cherry tomatoes, and sun-dried tomatoes directly on top of the cauliflower and cover without stirring. Season with pepper.

Cover and steam vegetables for 10 minutes.

Remove, cover, and serve the vegetables with the pine nuts and basil on top.

Serves 4

Grilled Romaine Salad

This knife-and-fork salad makes an impressive and quick light meal, or a great starter to a more elegant gathering. While you may never have thought to cook a salad, once you try this, you may be dreaming up other greens that can be cooked. This technique is also great for a unique twist on Caesar salad.

- 3 tablespoons olive oil
- 1 tablespoon Dijon mustard
- 1 teaspoon balsamic vinegar
- 4 heads romaine lettuce
- 4 tablespoons raw sunflower seeds
- Freshly ground black pepper, to taste

Preheat a gas or charcoal grill to medium heat.

In a small bowl, combine the olive oil, mustard, and vinegar. Brush the heads of lettuce with the oil mixture.

Lay the lettuce on the heated grill and cook until it starts to wilt and you can see grill marks.

Serve warm, topped with the sunflower seeds. Season with freshly ground black pepper and eat with a knife and fork.

Serves 4

Tomato-Stuffed Portobello Mushrooms

Grilling portobello mushrooms is nothing new, especially in the vegetarian world, but grilling and stuffing them? Now that's something you've got to try. With a flavorful filling of tomatoes and fresh herbs, this makes an impressive vegetarian dish that tastes as good as it looks.

- 2 portobello mushroom caps, gills and stems removed
- 2 tablespoons olive oil, divided
- 2 medium tomatoes, seeded and chopped
- 2 cloves garlic, minced
- ¼ cup fresh basil, chopped
- 2 tablespoons fresh rosemary, chopped
- 1 tablespoon balsamic vinegar
- Freshly ground black pepper, to taste

Heat a gas or charcoal grill over medium heat. Brush the mushrooms with half the olive oil and grill for 5 minutes per side.

In a medium bowl, combine the tomatoes, garlic, herbs, and vinegar. Season with freshly ground black pepper.

Make sure the mushrooms are top-side down on the grill. Carefully spoon the tomato mixture into the caps. Cover and cook for another minute.

Remove from grill and serve.

Serves 2

Spinach and Mushroom Soufflé

You may think of a soufflé as something fancy that is hard to make, but it's really not that difficult, and it makes an impressive dinner. This one has savory spinach and mushrooms, but feel free to customize it to your liking with whatever you have on hand. Even if your soufflé deflates after it comes out of the oven, it will still be delicious.

- 2 tablespoons olive oil
- 3 tablespoons almond flour
- 1 cup mushrooms, sliced
- 1 onion, chopped
- Freshly ground black pepper, to taste
- 2 cups almond milk
- 1 teaspoon arrowroot powder
- 6 large eggs, separated
- 2 cups baby spinach leaves

Preheat oven to 425 degrees F.

Spray the inside of a soufflé dish with cooking spray and coat with the almond flour.

Heat the 2 tablespoons of olive oil over medium heat in a large skillet and add the mushrooms and onions. Season with freshly ground black pepper. Cook until soft and lightly browned, set aside.

Heat the almond milk in a small saucepan, but don't boil. Add the arrowroot powder and whisk. Pour the milk mixture over the mushrooms. Allow to cool, then add the egg yolks.

Put the egg whites in a mixer and beat until stiff. Carefully fold the egg whites and spinach into the milk mixture. Pour into soufflé dish.

Bake for 40 minutes. Do not open the oven at all. Allow to rest for 5 minutes before serving.

Serves 4

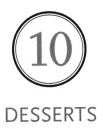

DESSERTS

Autumn Morning Muffins

These muffins are filled with the foods of the harvest—crisp, tart apples, cinnamon, and pumpkin. Almond meal and flaxseed flour replace white flour for a gluten-free baked good with a hearty, delicious flavor. Store flaxseed flour, which becomes rancid quickly, in a covered container in the refrigerator.

- 2 large eggs
- 1 cup pumpkin puree
- ½ cup applesauce
- ½ teaspoon vanilla
- 1¼ cups almond meal
- ¼ cup flaxseed flour
- 2 teaspoons baking powder

- ¼ teaspoon baking soda
- 1 teaspoon cinnamon
- ½ teaspoon ginger
- ½ teaspoon cloves
- ½ cup chopped walnuts
- 1 cup Granny Smith or McIntosh apples, peeled and chopped

Preheat oven to 350 degrees F. Combine the eggs, pumpkin puree, applesauce, and vanilla in a large mixing bowl. Sift the dry ingredients and add to the egg mixture. Fold gently to mix. Stir in the walnuts and the apples.

Bake for 20 to 30 minutes, or until browned and set. These muffins freeze beautifully for later use.

Serves 4

Caveman Custard

Custard is an old-fashioned sort of dish made from eggs and milk. This version is reinvented for the Paleo diet and uses almond milk and honey for flavor. Serve it with fresh fruit for a warm, comforting dessert on a cold winter day.

- 2 cups almond milk
- 6 large egg yolks
- 3 tablespoons honey

- 1 teaspoon cinnamon
- ½ teaspoon nutmeg
- 1 teaspoon vanilla extract

Preheat oven to 350 degrees F. Warm the almond milk in a saucepan until just simmering. Beat the egg yolks in a small mixing bowl. Slowly ladle half the almond milk into the eggs, a few drops at a time, vigorously whisking so the eggs don't cook.

Transfer the eggs and milk mixture to the saucepan and return to the heat. Add the remaining ingredients and cook over medium heat for 8 minutes, stirring constantly, until the custard thickens slightly.

Pour the custard into an ovenproof casserole dish. Set it in a baking pan and fill the pan with 2 inches of hot water. Slide the pan with the casserole dish carefully into the oven and cook for 30 minutes, or until the custard is set.

Serves 4

Baked Peaches

Peaches are high in sugar making them an infrequent indulgence on the Paleo diet, but when they're in season, it's hard to resist. Select peaches that give slightly to the touch and have a fresh aroma. The base color of the peach should be cream, not green. Green peaches were picked too early and will never be sweet.

- 4 ripe peaches, cut in half
- 3 tablespoons olive or coconut oil
- 2 tablespoons honey
- 1 teaspoon cinnamon
- ½ teaspoon almond extract

Preheat oven to 350 degrees F. Place the peaches on a baking sheet. Mix the remaining ingredients in a small bowl.

Fill the peach cavities with the mixture. Bake for 15 to 20 minutes, or until tender and juicy.

Serves 4

Berry Blitz

Berries are among the healthiest foods you can eat, and should be included several times each week on the Paleo diet. Use fresh berries when they are in season, or try frozen berries during the winter. Simply thaw them for 10 to 15 minutes on the counter.

- 1 cup strawberries, sliced
- 1 cup blueberries
- 1 cup raspberries
- 1 cup blackberries
- Juice and zest of 2 limes
- 2 tablespoons honey
- ¼ cup fresh mint leaves, chopped

Combine the fruit gently in a serving bowl. In a smaller bowl, mix the lime juice, zest, honey, and mint.

Pour the lime juice mixture over the fruit and mix gently to serve.

Serves 4

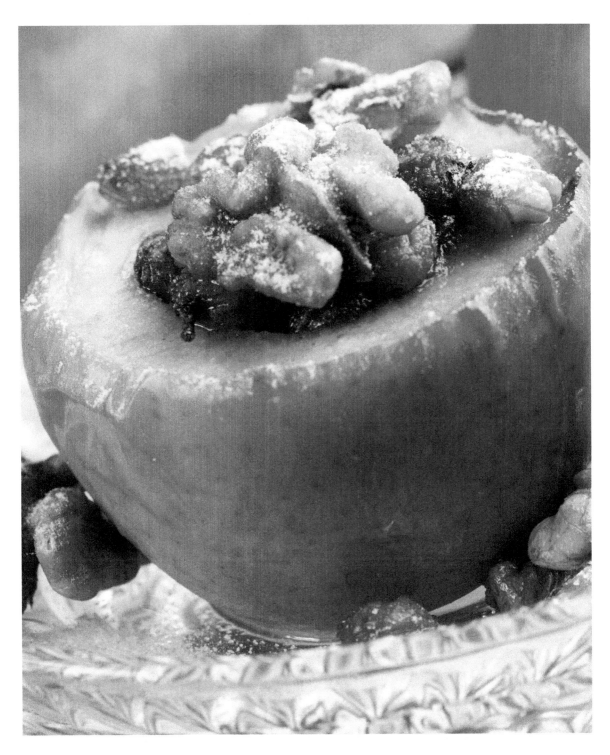

Baked Apples (page 298)

Baked Apples

You can treat these baked apples as either a dessert or a breakfast treat. You'll find the best cooking apples in mid to late fall. Choose tart but sweet varieties that have a firm texture. Try Winesap, Gravenstein, Jonagold, Fuji, or Pink Lady apples.

- 4 large baking apples
- Juice and zest of 1 lemon
- 3 tablespoons olive or coconut oil
- 3 tablespoons honey
- 1 teaspoon cinnamon
- ½ cup raisins
- ½ cup chopped walnuts

Preheat oven to 350 degrees F. Wash and core the apples.

Mix the remaining ingredients in a small bowl. Stuff the apples with the mixture.

Place the apples on a baking sheet and bake for 30 minutes, or until tender.

Serves 4

Melon Cooler

Honeydew melon is one of the sweetest melons and is delicious in smoothies and slushies. Buy several when they are in season, in mid to late summer, and freeze extra melon cubes for later. Honeydew melon is ripe when it exudes a sweet aroma and has a slightly fuzzy texture.

- 2 cups honeydew melon, cubed
- ½ cup lime juice
- 1 cup coconut water
- ½ cup ice cubes
- 1 teaspoon honey
- ¼ cup fresh mint leaves

Puree the melon cubes and the lime juice in a blender until smooth. Add the remaining ingredients and puree again.

Serves 4

Paleo Chocolate Chip Cookies

What kind of dessert section would this be without chocolate chip cookies? Not a very good one, if we do say so ourselves. This recipe does not adhere to super strict Paleo standards, but it is grain free and does not contain any refined sugar. Because of this, they may not be as sweet as you might be used to, but we think that once you try them, you'll realize that it's sweet enough for a satisfying treat on a special occasion—just the way a dessert should be.

- 3 cups almond flour
- 1 teaspoon baking soda
- 2 large eggs
- ¼ cup pure maple syrup
- 1 teaspoon pure vanilla extract
- ½ cup coconut oil
- 1 cup bittersweet chocolate chips

Preheat oven to 375 degrees F.

Sift together the dry ingredients in a medium mixing bowl. Beat in the eggs, maple syrup, vanilla, and coconut oil with a hand mixer until well combined.

Fold in the chocolate chips.

On a parchment-lined baking sheet, drop tablespoon-sized balls of cookie dough about 2 inches apart. Bake for 15 minutes. Remove from oven, cool, and serve.

Makes 2 dozen

Gingerbread Cookies

In this Paleo version of the classic spiced cookie, you're getting no refined sugar and no grains while enjoying a heavily spiced cookie that makes a perfect treat all year round. Molasses is the key to getting part of the classic flavor in these treats, but if you wish to skip it, you can use maple syrup instead.

- ¼ cup molasses
- 2 tablespoons pure maple syrup
- 3 tablespoons palm shortening
- 1 tablespoon coconut milk
- 3 cups almond flour
- 1 teaspoon cinnamon
- ½ teaspoon ground ginger
- ½ teaspoon ground cloves
- ¼ teaspoon ground nutmeg
- ½ teaspoon baking soda

Preheat oven to 350 degrees F.

Bring molasses to a boil in a small saucepan. Add the maple syrup, palm shortening, and coconut milk. Stir and remove from heat.

Combine the dry ingredients in a small bowl and pour the molasses mixture on top. Stir well.

Chill the dough for 20 minutes.

Roll the dough out to about a ¼-inch thickness. Using cookie cutters, cut out cookies and lay on a parchment-lined baking sheet.

Bake for 10 minutes, remove from oven, and cool. Decorate if you would like, or just serve and enjoy!

Makes 1 dozen

High Fiber Primal Cookies

These deliciously nutty cookies will remind you of your favorite oatmeal cookies, but to your surprise, there are no oats! Loaded with nuts, spices, and coconut, you'll enjoy the taste of these lightly sweetened cookies, but you won't miss any of the junk that is in packaged or high sugar varieties.

- 2 cups almond meal
- ½ cup ground flax seed
- ½ cup unsweetened, shredded coconut
- ½ cup raw sunflower seeds
- ½ cup raw pumpkin seeds
- 1 tablespoon cinnamon
- 1 teaspoon baking soda
- 2 large eggs
- 1 tablespoon pure vanilla extract
- ¼ cup pure maple syrup
- ½ cup coconut oil

Preheat oven to 325 degrees F.

In a large mixing bowl, sift the dry ingredients, including the seeds and coconut. In a separate bowl, combine the eggs, vanilla, maple syrup, and coconut oil.

Fold the wet ingredients into the dry and stir until well mixed. Drop the batter by the tablespoonful onto a parchment-lined baking sheet, approximately 2 inches apart.

Bake for 15 minutes, remove from oven, and cool completely before serving.

Makes 1 dozen

Raspberry Muffins

Raspberries add tart flavor and a chewy texture to these hearty muffins. Raspberries are in season in early summer, and again in fall. They are highly perishable, though, and should be refrigerated and stored within a day. Substitute frozen raspberries if you like, but don't thaw them before stirring them into the batter.

- 2 large eggs
- 3 ripe bananas, mashed
- ½ cup applesauce
- 1 teaspoon vanilla extract
- 1¼ cups almond meal

- 2 teaspoons baking powder
- ¼ teaspoon baking soda
- ¼ teaspoon cinnamon
- ¼ cup flaxseed flour
- 1 cup raspberries

Preheat oven to 350 degrees F. Spray a muffin pan with cooking spray.

Combine the eggs, banana, applesauce, and vanilla extract in a large mixing bowl. Add the dry ingredients and mix gently.

Fold in the raspberries gently. Pour ½ cup batter in each muffin cup. Bake 20 to 30 minutes, or until browned.

Serves 6

Peach Slushy

Nothing says summer like peaches. Peach ice cream, peach cobbler, and peaches and cream all are sweet treats that bring out the glorious flavor of in-season peaches. This peach slushy makes a delicious summer breakfast and tastes like peach ice cream. Make several bags and keep them in your freezer for a quick breakfast.

- 8 ripe peaches, peeled, pitted, and cubed
- 1 cup almond milk
- 1 cup full-fat coconut milk
- ½ teaspoon vanilla
- 3 tablespoons honey

Combine all the ingredients in a large mixing bowl. Ladle the mixture into plastic quart freezer bags or small freezer-safe containers.

Freeze the mixture overnight, or until firm. To serve, thaw the mixture on the counter for 30 minutes. Scoop the mixture into glasses and enjoy.

Serves 4

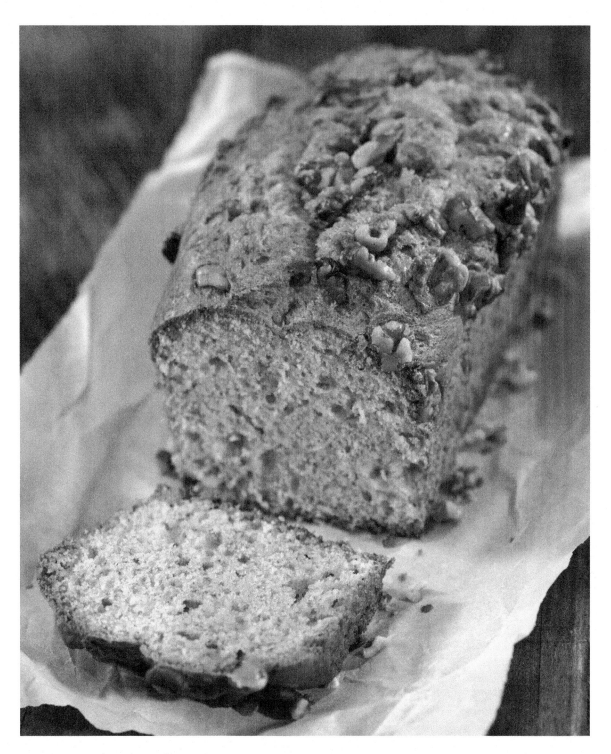

Banana Bread (page 306)

Banana Bread

Believe it or not, this loaf is baked without grains or wheat, and without sugar. Instead, the sweetness comes from very ripe bananas. When your banana skins are almost entirely black, that's when you know they'll be good in this recipe. While this is still not something you want to eat every single day, you can indulge in this tasty treat once in awhile without guilt.

- 3 cups almond flour
- 2 teaspoons baking soda
- 1 tablespoon cinnamon
- ¼ cup coconut oil
- 4 large eggs
- 2 large, very ripe bananas
- 1 tablespoon pure vanilla extract
- ½ cup walnuts, chopped and toasted

Preheat oven to 350 degrees F.

Sift the almond flour, baking soda, and cinnamon in a bowl. Add the rest of the ingredients and stir well to combine.

Pour the batter into a loaf pan greased with coconut oil. Bake for 25 to 28 minutes, until toothpick inserted in the center comes out clean.

Cool completely, remove from pan, and slice.

Serves 8 to 10

Flourless Chocolate Delight

This is a deep and rich chocolate cake that will satisfy even the most intense cravings. There's no sugar besides what's in the chocolate, so it's got a deep chocolate flavor that's not super sweet like many desserts you may be used to. Use the best quality chocolate you can afford and stick to one that is 72- to 85-percent cocoa for the best results—not to mention the least sugar!

- 7 large eggs
- 14 ounces bittersweet chocolate, chopped
- 14 tablespoons coconut oil
- ¼ cup strong brewed coffee
- 1 teaspoon pure vanilla extract

Preheat oven to 325 degrees F.

Grease a 9-inch springform pan with oil. Wrap the bottom of the pan in foil.

Beat the eggs with a mixer for about 7 minutes, until frothy and doubled in volume.

Melt the chocolate and remaining oil in either a double boiler or the microwave, stirring frequently to avoid burning. Add the coffee and vanilla.

Carefully fold the chocolate into the eggs and spread the batter in the prepared pan.

Put the pan in a large casserole or roasting pan and pour boiling water in the pan, filling halfway up the sides of the springform pan.

Bake for 18 minutes and insert an instant read thermometer in the center. When it reaches 140 degrees F, the cake is done.

Allow the cake to cool completely before removing the sides of the pan.

Cut into slices and serve.

Serves 8

Berry Tart

When making a dish that relies extensively on the flavor of berries—as this one does—it is best to wait until you can get the freshest and ripest berries possible. Not only will they be sweet enough that you won't need to add any sugar, but their flavor will be fresh and pronounced. If you must use out-of-season berries, you can add a tablespoon or so of honey to the berry mixture.

Filling:
- 4 cups fresh mixed berries of your choice
- 1 cup water
- Juice of 1 lemon

Crust:
- 1½ cups almond flour
- ¼ teaspoon baking soda
- ½ teaspoon cinnamon
- ¼ teaspoon nutmeg
- ¼ cup coconut oil
- 1 teaspoon pure vanilla extract

Preheat oven to 350 degrees F.

Heat berries, water, and lemon juice in a medium saucepan. Simmer for 15 minutes, stirring and mashing berries periodically.

While fruit is simmering, combine all ingredients for the crust together in a large bowl. When you have a stiff dough, press into a pie pan and bake for 10 minutes. Remove from oven and allow to cool for 5 minutes.

Add the berry mixture to the crust and refrigerate for 1 hour before serving.

Serves 6

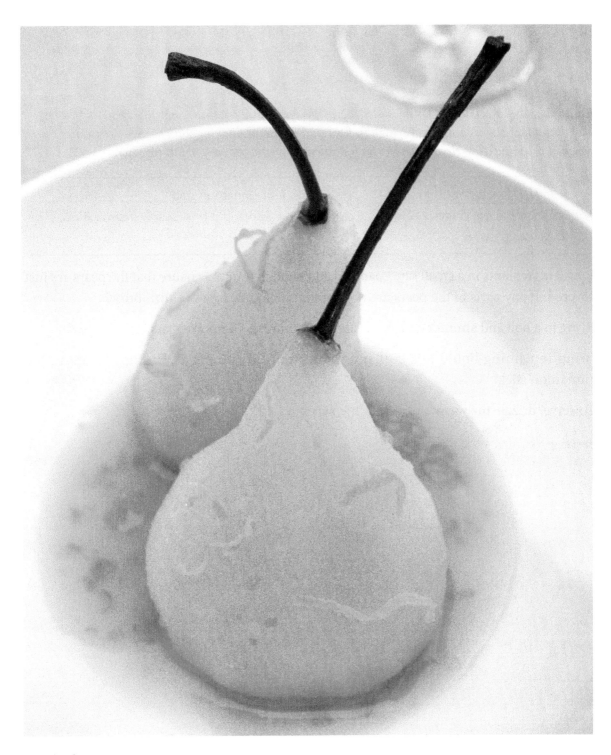

Poached Pears (page 310)

Poached Pears

Fruit makes a perfect dessert for the Paleo diet. It's sweet, but its natural sugar isn't bad for you the way that added sugars are. It's also high in fiber and nutrients, making it an even better choice. These poached pears make an elegant dessert for a dinner party and are easy to put together.

- Juice from 4 large oranges
- 1 small piece ginger, peeled
- 4 whole cloves
- 1 cinnamon stick
- 4 ripe but firm pears, such as Bosc, peeled and cored

Put all ingredients in a small saucepan and add enough water to ensure that the pears are just covered. If any parts of the pears are not covered in liquid, they will turn brown.

Bring to a boil and simmer on low for about 30 minutes. Remove pears.

Bring remaining liquid to a boil and reduce until it is thick and syrupy. Remove the cinnamon stick.

To serve, drizzle the warm pears with the syrup.

Serves 4

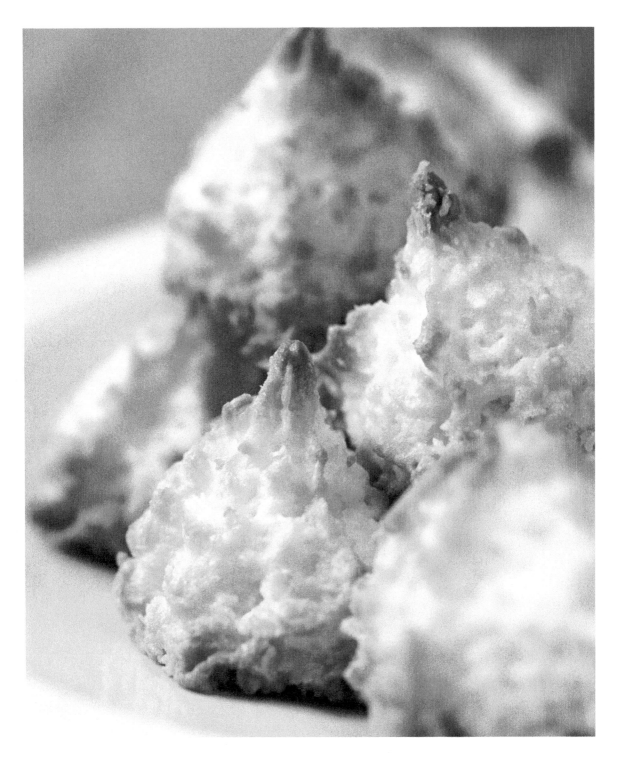

Coconut Macaroons (page 312)

Coconut Macaroons

With only a few ingredients, these coconut treats are lightly sweet and surprisingly easy to whip up. Make sure to use unsweetened coconut so that you get the best flavor, and also no refined sugar. With hints of vanilla, these will bring a taste of the tropics to the end of your meal.

- 6 large egg whites
- ¼ cup pure maple syrup
- 1 teaspoon pure vanilla extract
- 3 cups shredded, unsweetened coconut

Preheat oven to 325 degrees F.

Beat the egg whites in a stand mixer until they form stiff peaks. Gently fold in the maple syrup, vanilla, and coconut.

Form into 1-inch balls and put on a parchment-lined baking sheet. Bake for 15 to 17 minutes, or until lightly browned.

Cool before serving.

Makes 1 dozen

Primal Brownies

Like many of the dessert recipes you'll find here, these brownies are a better version of the classic dessert they're modeled after. They are more rich than sweet, and while they don't follow the Paleo principle strictly to the letter, they are close enough that we think they fit. As long as you don't eat the whole pan (it will be difficult!), you should be able to enjoy one of these every now and then without the guilt and remorse that comes with eating the real thing.

- 1 cup coconut oil
- 5 ounces bittersweet chocolate
- ½ cup pure maple syrup
- ¼ cup unsweetened cocoa powder
- 4 large eggs
- 1 teaspoon baking soda
- 1 tablespoon pure vanilla extract
- 1 cup raw, unsalted almond butter
- ¼ cup coconut flour

Preheat oven to 350 degrees F.

Mix the coconut oil, bittersweet chocolate, and maple syrup in a small saucepan over low heat. When melted and combined, remove from heat.

Add in the cocoa powder, stir, and set aside.

With a wooden spoon, blend in the eggs, baking soda, and vanilla. Add in the almond butter and stir until combined.

Fold in the coconut flour.

Pour batter into a 9 x 13-inch baking dish that has been lightly greased with coconut oil. Bake for 30 minutes.

Cool completely before cutting and serving.

Makes 1 dozen brownies

Chocolate Almond Butter Candies

If you are in the camp that loves those chocolate peanut butter cups (and who isn't?), then you'll love these delightful candies that adhere surprisingly well to the Paleo plan. While they aren't nearly as sweet as what they are modeled after, they are surprisingly satisfying and, with only two ingredients, they don't have any of the bad stuff you get from the store-bought variety. Make sure that the almond butter you use for these contains only almonds.

• 1 cup bittersweet chocolate chips	• ½ cup natural almond butter

Melt the chocolate chips on low heat, either in the microwave or on the stove in a double boiler, being extra careful not to burn them.

Using a clean pastry brush, paint the chocolate into candy molds or ice cube trays. Put in the freezer for 10 minutes.

Remove tray from freezer and quickly fill each mold with almond butter. Using the pastry brush again, paint over the tops with the almond butter.

Return to the freezer for 10 more minutes. When the candies are completely hardened, pop out and serve.

Makes 10

Pecan Bark

Roasted and salted nuts go perfectly with the deep, intense flavor of dark chocolate, and you're sure to love this easy-to-make bark. Use any variety of nuts you like, or even a mixture, if the mood strikes. Either way, you'll love these sweet and salty treats.

- 12 ounces dark chocolate, chopped
- 1 cup roasted pecans

Melt the chocolate in a double boiler or in the microwave, being extra careful not to burn it.

Stir in the nuts and spread the mixture on a parchment-lined baking sheet.

Freeze until solid and break into chunks.

Makes about 1 pound

Chocolate-Banana Milkshake

This can be a lot of things: an energizing breakfast, a quick snack to pick you up in the middle of the day, or a filling lunch replacement when you're in a hurry. We like it as a dessert, however, as it is sweet and chocolaty, and a great after-dinner delight. With no added sugar, it comes together fast and satisfies any craving you may have for chocolate or ice cream.

- 1 cup unsweetened almond milk
- 1 tablespoon natural peanut butter
- 3 tablespoons unsweetened cocoa powder
- 1 large banana
- 1 cup ice

Put all ingredients in a blender in the order listed. Blend until smooth and creamy and serve with a straw.

Serves 1

SNACKS AND BEVERAGES

Caveman Trail Mix

Trail mix is full of antioxidants and protein for energy, making it a great on-the-go breakfast for the Paleo dieter. Substitute your favorite combination of nuts and dried fruit, and pack it in individual bags to grab quickly on busy mornings. Trail mix makes a great post-workout or sports practice food, too.

- 2 cups shredded coconut flakes
- ½ cup dried apricots, apples, blueberries, goji berries, or cherries, or a combination
- ½ cup chopped pecans, walnuts, or macadamia nuts
- ¼ cup cacao

Combine all ingredients in a large mixing bowl. Store in an airtight container for up to one month.

Serves 4

Nutty Apple Snacks

Sometimes you don't have time for a sit-down lunch. This recipe is the perfect solution to a frenzied schedule. Nut butter and chopped nuts provide energy-boosting protein, while the fruit provides a satisfying crunch. Select tart, but sweet apples with a firm texture.

- 2 apples, any variety
- ½ cup almond butter
- 1 tablespoon honey
- Juice and zest of 1 orange
- ½ teaspoon pure vanilla extract
- ½ teaspoon cinnamon
- ⅛ cup walnuts or pecans, chopped
- ⅛ cup pumpkin seeds

Cut the apples into quarters. Remove the seeds but leave the peels. Mix the remaining ingredients together in a bowl.

Spread the almond butter mixture on the apples for a quick, but satisfying lunch. This spread packs well to take on outings or for travel.

Serves 4

Chunky Applesauce

Apple season calls to mind crisp fall days, warm, wooly sweaters, and the smell of cinnamon and cloves. This chunky applesauce is the epitome of fall and will warm you on a chilly day. Top it with dried fruit for a quick, but satisfying snack. Select several varieties of apples for an added depth of flavor.

• 8 tart baking apples	• 1 teaspoon cinnamon
• Juice and zest from 1 lemon	• ½ teaspoon nutmeg
• Juice and zest from 1 orange	• ½ teaspoon cloves
• 3 tablespoons honey	• 4 tablespoons olive or coconut oil

Peel, core and quarter the apples. Place them in a large saucepan with 1 inch of water. Cover the pan with the lid and simmer over medium-low heat for 30 minutes, or until tender.

Transfer the apples to a blender or food processor, and blend them until they are almost smooth, with a few chunks remaining.

Return the apple puree to the saucepan. Add the remaining ingredients and simmer for 20 minutes.

Serves 4

Homemade Fruit Rollups

These fruit rollups are not the chemical-laden ones you may be used to in the grocery store. Instead, they are made with real fruit, and while they take a while to make and require a dehydrator, they can satisfy a craving that a real piece of fruit may not be able to. Great for kids as well.

- 2 apples, any type
- 1 pint strawberries, stemmed
- ¼ cup purified water
- 1 teaspoon cinnamon

Preheat oven to 200 degrees F. Peel, core and dice apples.

Add apples, strawberries, water, and cinnamon in a blender and process about 30 seconds, or until smooth.

Pour mixture on a parchment-lined baking sheet and place in a dehydrator.

Dehydrate for 6 to 8 hours. Remove sheet and flip fruit. Continue drying another 4 to 6 hours.

Serves 6

Ants on a Log

This is a classic snack that is easy to make and totally nutritious. Almond butter replaces the peanut butter for a different take, and you can use raisins, currants, or whatever dried fruit you like.

- 2 celery stalks
- 4 tablespoons almond butter
- ¼ cup dried raisins or cranberries

Spread almond butter on each celery stalk. Add the fruit to the top.

Serve and enjoy!

Serves 2

Dates Wrapped in Bacon

These easy-to-make snacks are a great combination of salty, sweet, and crunchy, and they fit in the Paleo plan well because it's hard to get this combo elsewhere. These make a great anytime snack or an easy appetizer when you're looking for something quick.

- 8 slices uncured, nitrate-free bacon
- 16 medium dates
- 16 raw almonds

Cook bacon over medium-low heat until almost crisp, being careful not to make it too crispy. Remove from pan and allow to cool.

Stuff each date with an almond, and wrap with half of a bacon slice. Use a toothpick to secure if making for an appetizer.

Serve warm.

Serves 4

Coconut Almond Butter Bananas

These are a fast and easy treat that anyone can make at any time. Between the banana and the almond butter, you're getting plenty of fiber and protein, while eating something that seems much more decadent than it really is.

- 1 large banana
- 2 tablespoons almond butter
- 2 tablespoons coconut milk
- 1 tablespoon shredded unsweetened coconut
- 1 tablespoon almonds, sliced

Slice banana and put in a bowl. Top with almond butter and coconut milk. Garnish with the shredded coconut and sliced almonds. Eat with a spoon and enjoy!

Serves 1

Paleo Spiced Nuts

Nuts are a great snack when on the Paleo diet, but sometimes you want something more interesting than plain-old roasted nuts. These crunchy and toasty morsels fit the bill perfectly. Use any combination of nuts you like or have on hand—what's in the recipe is just a suggestion. Make sure that whatever you use is raw and unsalted.

- ½ cup whole almonds
- ½ cup walnuts
- ¼ cup sunflower seeds
- ¼ cup pumpkin seeds
- ¼ cup pecans, chopped
- ¼ cup pistachios
- 1 teaspoon dried rosemary
- 1 teaspoon dried thyme
- ¼ teaspoon cayenne pepper
- 1 tablespoon olive oil

Preheat oven to 350 degrees F.

Put everything in a gallon-size freezer bag. Shake to make sure all nuts are coated thoroughly with the oil and spices.

Lay on a parchment-lined baking sheet in an even layer and bake for 12 to 15 minutes, or until nuts are toasted. Cool completely before serving.

Makes 2 cups

Brussels Sprouts Chips

Even if you don't like Brussels sprouts, you'll probably love these chips, for two reasons. First of all, roasted sprouts don't have that sulfurous odor and flavor that comes from steaming. Second, these are actually crunchy and chip-like, but they are healthier than anything you're going to get out of a bag. Use only the outer leaves from the Brussels sprouts and don't bother with any that are wilted.

- 2 cups Brussels sprout leaves
- 2 tablespoons olive oil
- Freshly ground black pepper, to taste

Preheat oven to 350 degrees F. Toss the leaves with the olive oil and season with pepper if you'd like.

Lay in a single layer on a parchment-lined baking sheet, using two sheets or working in batches, if necessary.

Bake for about 10 minutes, until the leaves are browned and crispy. Allow to cool and serve.

Makes 2 cups

Turkey Avocado Rollups

Finding healthy and easy snacks is difficult no matter what kind of diet you're on. While you have lots of options on the Paleo plan, sometimes you need something that is similar to a meal, but not huge. These rollups are almost like eating a turkey and avocado sandwich.

- 1 ripe avocado, peeled and pitted
- 1 tablespoon lemon juice
- 4 cherry tomatoes, roughly chopped
- Freshly ground black pepper, to taste
- 4 slices thick-cut turkey breast

Put the avocado and lemon juice in a bowl and mash thoroughly with a fork. Gently add in the tomatoes. Season with freshly ground black pepper.

Spread the avocado mixture on the turkey slices and roll up. Serve and enjoy!

Serves 1

Herbed Crackers

If you're craving something crunchy to eat, these easy herbed crackers will do the trick—and yes, they do fit on the Paleo diet. Made with ground nuts instead of wheat flour, they are great for anyone who is on a gluten-free diet, but still misses crackers or chips.

- 2 cups almond meal
- 2 tablespoons Italian seasoning
- 2 tablespoons water
- 1 large egg white
- 1 tablespoon olive oil
- Freshly ground black pepper, to taste

Preheat oven to 350 degrees F.

In a medium bowl, sift together the almond meal and spices. Stir in the water, egg white, and olive oil. Using your hands, form into a stiff dough.

Roll out to about ⅛-inch thickness. Using a pairing knife, cut into 2-inch squares. Sprinkle lightly with fresh ground pepper.

Transfer the squares to a parchment-lined baking sheet and bake for 10 minutes until golden.

Let cool completely and serve.

Makes about 2 dozen

Crispy Pepperoni Bites

Once you try these, you'll realize that you can in fact live without pizza on the Paleo diet. Use any kind of toppings you want, and if you're feeling especially indulgent, you can even add a bit of cheese (although you can easily forgo it!). These are a quick and easy snack that will surely become one of your favorites.

- 12 slices high quality pepperoni
- ¼ cup marinara sauce
- Pizza toppings of your choice, such as olives, onions, peppers, or mushrooms

Preheat oven to 400 degrees F.

Lay pepperoni on a parchment-lined sheet tray and bake for 7 to 8 minutes, flipping them over halfway through.

While they are in the oven, take the time to make sure toppings are minced into tiny pieces.

Remove the pan from the oven and add sauce and desired toppings. Put it back in the oven and bake for 4 more minutes.

Serve warm and crispy, right from the oven.

Makes 1 dozen

Grill-Out Burger Bites

These burgers are so flavorful that you won't miss the buns. Serve these with sweet potato fries for a Paleo-style cookout.

- 1 pound grass-fed ground beef
- ½ teaspoon minced garlic
- ⅛ cup red onion, finely minced
- 1 can roasted green chilies
- 2 strips uncured, nitrate-free bacon, cooked and crumbled
- 1 large egg, beaten
- Freshly ground black pepper, to taste

Combine the ingredients in a large mixing bowl, using your fingers to thoroughly mix them.

Form the mixture into 2- to 4-inch rounds. Grill for 15 to 20 minutes, flipping halfway through the cooking time. The burgers are done when flecks of gray fat appear on the meat.

Serves 4

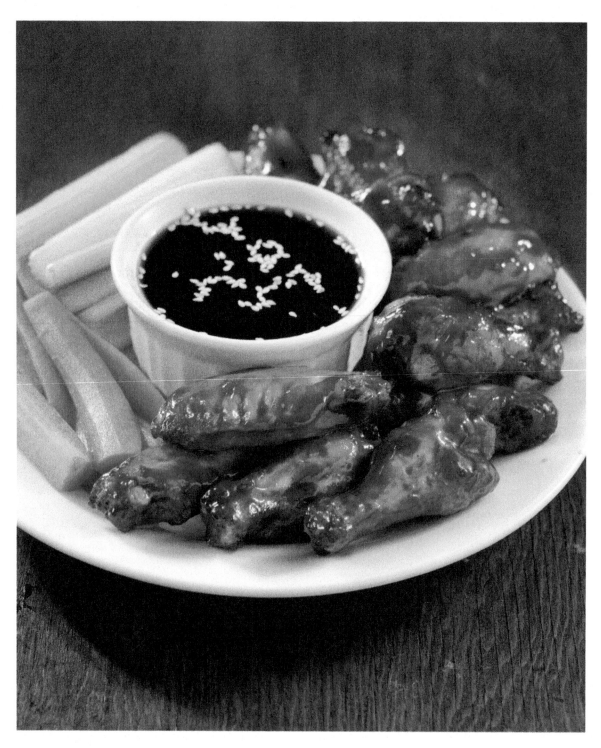

Teriyaki Chicken Drumsticks

Teriyaki Chicken Drumsticks

Toss this simple dish in your slow cooker in the morning, and by dinner, you'll have tender, flavorful, Asian-inspired chicken that the whole family will love. Substitute whole, cut-up chicken for the drumsticks if you prefer.

- 8 chicken drumsticks
- ½ cup orange juice
- ½ cup coconut aminos
- ½ teaspoon ginger
- ½ teaspoon garlic
- Freshly ground black pepper, to taste

Place the drumsticks in the slow cooker and turn the slow cooker to low. Combine the remaining ingredients in a small bowl. Pour this mixture over the drumsticks. Cover and cook for 5 to 6 hours, or until tender. Turn occasionally so the chicken is thoroughly coated with the sauce.

Serves 4

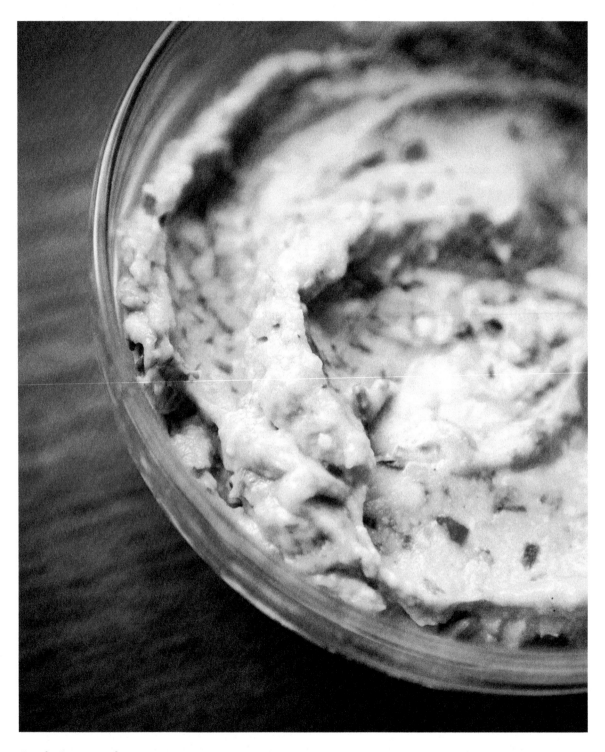

Fresh Guacamole

Fresh Guacamole

This easy, crowd-pleasing dip is one that is healthy as long as you don't eat it with a bunch of fried chips. Instead, try it with some veggies—peppers, celery, carrots, and cucumbers work well. If you're going to store it, squeeze some more lime juice over the top before putting in the refrigerator to keep it from browning.

- 2 ripe avocados, peeled and pitted
- 1 medium tomato, seeded and chopped
- ½ small red onion, diced
- 2 tablespoons fresh cilantro, chopped
- 1 clove garlic, minced
- Freshly ground black pepper, to taste
- Juice of 1 lime

In a medium bowl, mash the avocados with a fork until creamy, leaving as few chunks as possible.

Add in the tomatoes, onions, cilantro, and garlic. Season with freshly ground black pepper. Stir gently to combine and add the lime juice. Serve immediately.

Serves 6 to 8

Caveman Hummus

While hummus is traditionally made with chickpeas—a strict no-no on the Paleo diet—this version is made with zucchini. It's still creamy and delicious, and it's likely your guests won't know they aren't getting all those extra carbs.

- 2 medium zucchini
- ¾ cup tahini
- ¼ cup olive oil
- Juice of 2 lemons
- 2 garlic cloves, minced
- 1 tablespoon ground cumin
- Freshly ground black pepper, to taste
- Veggies, such as sliced bell peppers, tomatoes, carrots, and cucumbers, for serving

Peel and chop the zucchini and put in a food processor. Process until smooth.

Add the tahini, olive oil, lemon juice, garlic, and cumin and puree until creamy smooth. Season with freshly ground black pepper. Serve with sliced veggies for dipping.

Serves 6 to 8

Herbed Grilled Olives

Olives are high in good-for-you fat, and are a flavorful appetizer. While they are good on their own, tossing them with some herbs and garlic before throwing them on a hot grill makes them extra special— perfect for some quick finger-food before a Mediterranean-themed dinner.

- 1 cup whole-oil packed olives, mixed
- 1 tablespoon fresh rosemary, chopped
- 1 tablespoon fresh oregano, chopped
- 1 clove garlic, minced
- Freshly ground black pepper, to taste

Toss the olives with the herbs and garlic. Season with freshly ground black pepper.

Heat a gas or charcoal grill over medium heat. Put olives in a grill basket and heat for 6 to 8 minutes, turning to make sure they are evenly heated.

Put in a warmed dish and serve immediately.

Serves 4

Bacon-Wrapped Scallops

This is a super fast and easy appetizer that many people love. Make sure to buy the larger sea scallops for best presentation, and if you can get them dry packed, you'll save yourself some sodium and they'll brown better.

- 1 pound uncured, nitrate-free, thick-cut bacon strips
- 18 bay scallops, rinsed
- Freshly ground black pepper, to taste
- Smoked paprika

Preheat oven to 400 degrees F. Cut bacon strips in half and wrap around the scallops. Secure with toothpicks. Season with freshly ground black pepper.

Lay on a baking sheet and sprinkle with paprika. Bake for 15 minutes, flip and bake for 15 more minutes until browned. Serve immediately.

Serves 6

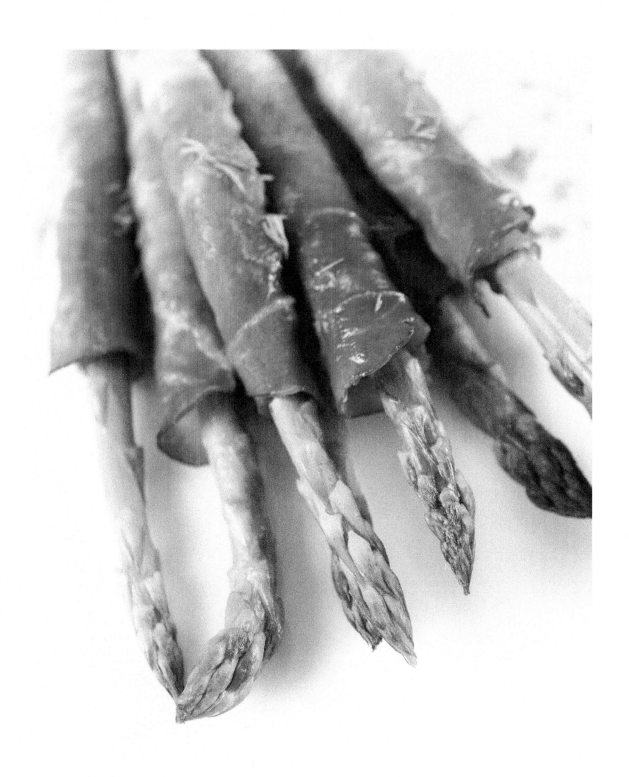

Prosciutto-Wrapped Asparagus (page 338)

Prosciutto-Wrapped Asparagus

This is an easy appetizer that comes together fast. These work well for everything from casual gatherings to fancy dinner parties, and your guests are sure to love them. Get the highest quality prosciutto you can afford for the best flavor.

- 1 pound asparagus spears
- ¼ pound prosciutto, thinly sliced
- ½ medium onion, thinly sliced
- Freshly ground black pepper, to taste

Preheat oven to 400 degrees F. Slice the asparagus into 4-inch pieces.

Lay the prosciutto slices on a sheet pan and lay a few onion slices and asparagus pieces on each slice. Season with freshly ground black pepper. Roll them up, tucking the flap down.

Serves 8

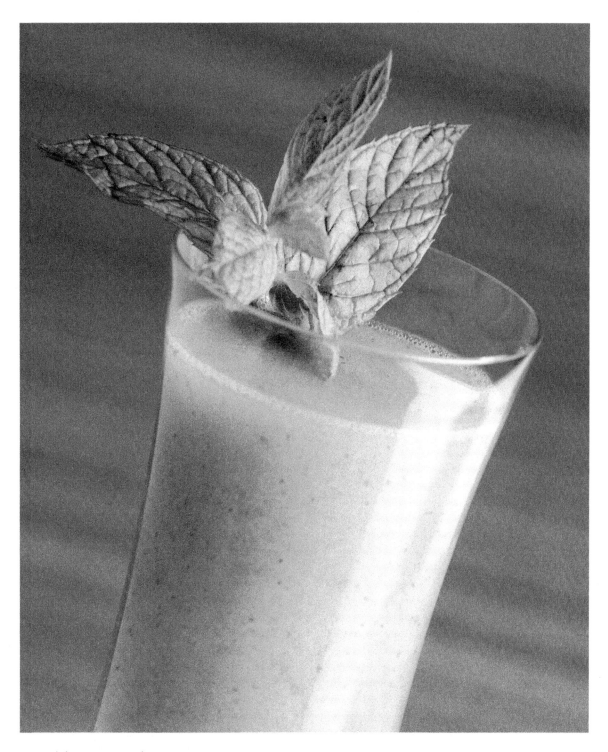

Energizing Green Juice (page 340)

Energizing Green Juice

While fruit juice is prohibited on the Paleo diet, juicing your own fruits and vegetables is different than buying processed juice. This drink is refreshing, high in vitamins and minerals, and easy to prepare if you have a juicer. While you still don't want to drink too much of it, it's a great drink when you're tired of drinking water.

- 1 cucumber
- 1 Granny Smith apple
- 1 celery stalk
- 1 kiwi
- Small bunch fresh mint

Put all ingredients in a juicer, pour into glasses, and serve chilled.

Serves 2

Homemade Almond Milk

Almond milk is a great alternative to traditional dairy, and this easy homemade version is deliciously creamy and satisfying. This is a basic recipe, but you can customize it to your tastes by adding dates for sweetness or a little vanilla extract for flavor. This makes a great warm drink before bed at night.

- 1 cup raw almonds
- 3 cups water, plus more for covering

Cover the almonds in water and allow to soak for 6 to 8 hours or overnight.

Drain the water and put the almonds in a blender with 3 cups fresh water. Blend until smooth.

Pour the liquid through a cheesecloth and store in the refrigerator. This will keep for 3 to 4 days.

Makes 2 cups

Citrus Cooler

This bright and citrusy drink is easy to make and comes together fast. It's a great addition to breakfast instead of packaged orange juice or other juices that are loaded with artificial flavorings and chemicals. This also makes a great meal replacement in the morning or afternoon. For more fiber, add some ground flax seed before blending.

- 1 cup cold water
- 1 ruby red grapefruit, peeled, white pith removed
- 1 large orange, peeled
- 1 cup frozen pineapple

Put all ingredients in a blender and blend on high until smooth and creamy. Serve immediately.

Serves 2

Paleo Hot Chocolate

While you may think of dairy when you think of hot cocoa, it doesn't have to be made with cow's milk and white sugar to be good. This version is made with almond milk, cocoa powder, and just enough honey to take away the bitterness of the cocoa. Serve this on a cold winter's day and no one—not even the youngest of the bunch—will complain, as it's just as rich and chocolaty as any dairy version you've ever had.

- 2 cups unsweetened almond milk
- 2 tablespoons unsweetened cocoa powder
- 1 teaspoon honey

Bring the cocoa powder and almond milk to a simmer, whisking constantly. Add the honey and pour into mugs.

Serve hot.

Serves 2

Chai Tea

This delicately spiced "tea" has a warm and comforting aroma that is perfect for a pick-me-up on a cold day. While there are many varieties of chai at the grocery store, this homemade version has a more complex and interesting flavor profile.

- 4 cups water
- 1 large piece fresh ginger, peeled and sliced
- 8 cardamom pods, cracked
- 1 bay leaf
- 4 whole peppercorns
- 1 tablespoon pure vanilla extract
- ½ teaspoon fennel seeds
- 4 whole cloves

Put all ingredients in a pot and bring to a boil. Cover and simmer for at least 20 minutes—longer if you like a stronger flavor.

Strain the tea through a strainer or cheesecloth. Pour into mugs and serve hot.

Serves 2

Cranberry Tea

Most people probably have images of white tea bags with the string on them when they think of hot tea, but the truth is that you can make your own tea by simply simmering your favorite herbs and spices in some hot water and then straining it. This version has a strong cranberry flavor along with spiciness that is perfect for a winter celebration.

- ¼ cup fresh cranberries
- 1 teaspoon honey
- 4 cups water
- 1 cinnamon stick
- 2 whole cloves
- ¼ cup orange juice

Put the cranberries, honey, and water in a medium saucepan and bring to a boil. Reduce heat and simmer for 10 minutes or until cranberries pop.

Add the rest of the ingredients and simmer for 10 more minutes. Strain through a strainer or cheesecloth and serve hot.

Serves 2

Paleo "Coffee"

While this may not be exactly the same as coffee, you may be surprised at how close it is. You may have to go to a health food store to get the ingredients, but if you're someone who relies on their daily java, this may be just the substitute you are looking for.

- 2 cups water
- 1 tablespoon roasted chicory root
- 1 tablespoon dried dandelion root
- 2 cardamom pods, cracked

Put all ingredients in a medium saucepan. Bring to a boil and reduce to a simmer. Simmer for 10 minutes.

Strain through a strainer or cheesecloth. Serve hot and enjoy!

Serves 2

CPSIA information can be obtained
at www.ICGtesting.com
Printed in the USA
BVOW07*1026070416
443248BV00032B/12/P

9 781623 152079